W9-CKL-747

DATE DUE

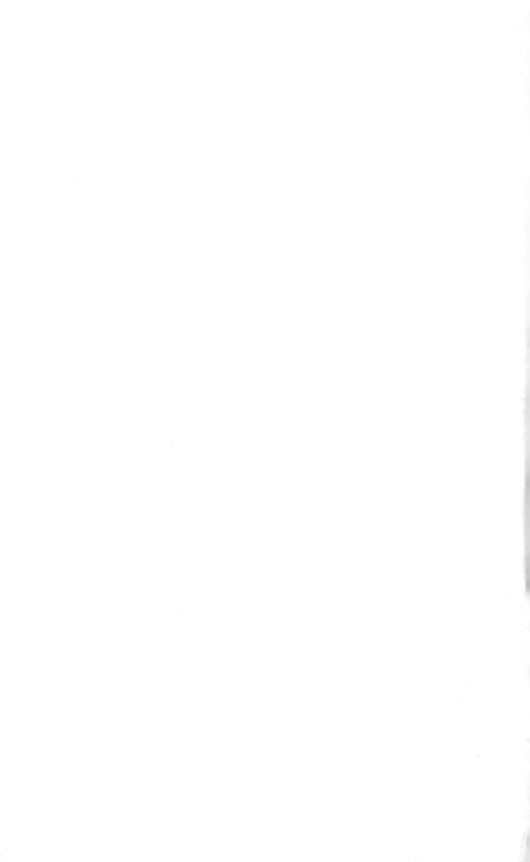

Springer Series: THE TEACHING OF NURSING

Series Editor: Diane O. McGivern, RN, PhD, FAAN

Barbara Stevens Barnum, RN, PhD, FAAN, consultant and author, was a professor of the Columbia University School of Nursing Division, New York City, and editor, *Nursing Leadership Forum,* until her retirement from these positions in 1998. Previously, she held appointments as editor of *Nursing & Health Care,* the journal of the National League for Nursing, and as director, Division of Health Services, Sciences and Education at Teachers College, Columbia University, where she held the Stewart Chair in the Department of Nursing Education, and, for part of her tenure, the chairmanship of the Department of Nursing Education.

Before coming to New York, Dr. Barnum coordinated the Nursing Service Administration Program of the College of Nursing, University of Illinois in Chicago, served as director of Nursing Staff Development at the University of Chicago Hospitals and Clinics, and held chief executive positions in both nursing practice and nursing education at Augustana Hospital and Health Care Center in Chicago.

Dr. Barnum has written widely in areas of nursing management, theory, and education. Her books include: *Nursing Theory: Analysis, Application, Evaluation* (5th ed.); *Spirituality in Nursing: From Traditional to New Age; The Nurse As Executive* (4th ed.), (with K. Kerfoot); and *Writing and Getting Published: A Primer for Nurses.*

A fellow in the American Academy of Nursing, Dr. Barnum has done extensive national and international consultation and continuing education, including an eight-year term as consultant to the Air Force Surgeon General and work in Germany, Norway, Australia, New Zealand, Japan, and Canada. Dr. Barnum presently writes and consults in areas of complementary medicine and spirituality.

Teaching Nursing in the Era of Managed Care

Barbara Stevens Barnum
RN, PhD, FAAN

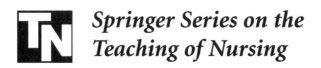

Springer Series on the
Teaching of Nursing

Springer Publishing Company, Inc.
536 Broadway
New York, NY 10012-3955

Acquisitions Editor: Ruth Chasek
Production Editor: Helen Song
Cover design by Janet Joachim

99 00 01 02 03 / 5 4 3 2 1

Library of Congress Cataloging-in-Publication-Data

Barnum, Barbara Stevens.
    Teaching nursing in the era of managed care / by Barbara Stevens Barnum.
        p.   cm. — (Teaching of nursing)
    Includes bibliographical references and index.
    ISBN 0-8261-1254-4
    1. Nursing—Study and teaching.   2. Nursing—Effect of managed care on.   3. Medical education.   4. Managed care plans (Medical care).   I. Title.   II. Series.
    [DNLM: 1. Education, Nursing.   2. Managed Care Programs—United States.   WY 18 B2635t   1999]
RT73.B27   1999
610.73'071'1—dc21
DNLM/DLC
for Library of Congress   98-37684
                                                                      CIP

Printed in the United States of America

Contents

Acknowledgments

This book is based on a series of lessons prepared for The Teagle Foundation as part of a comprehensive course on managed care, a combined effort of the Schools of Nursing of Vanderbilt University and Columbia University. Portions of the volume are tentatively scheduled to be available in 1999 on the Internet for college credit through the School of Nursing, Vanderbilt University. The grant, entitled, *To Support the Development and Piloting of the Advanced Practice Nursing Institute on Managed Care for Nurse Faculty*, was supported by The Teagle Foundation, a private foundation incorporated in Connecticut, established in 1944 by Walter C. Teagle, long-time president and later chairman of the board of Standard Oil Company, now Exxon Corporation. I wish to thank the Foundation for allowing this component of the grant to be published as a book.

I also wish to thank the Teagle Grant Advisory Board for their invaluable suggestions for improving the content of this material. Those members were: Ms. Lenore Appenzeller, Dr. Eleanor Barba, Dr. Cynthia Mersmann, Ms. Josephine Sapp, Dr. Mary Crabtree Tonges, and Ms. Norma Turini. I also wish to thank Dr. Roxane Spitzer, my project codirector from the Vanderbilt site. Dr. Spitzer and her staff were responsible for the many "bells and whistles"—the audiovisual displays that make the Internet version so attractive. She also prepared much grant material specific to explaining managed care.

Introduction

The purpose of this book is to reflect on how the system of managed care changes, or should change, a nursing faculty's practice and role function. The book is designed to help the nursing faculty member think through the changes in the health care delivery system resulting from the introduction of managed care. The objective of this exercise is to ensure that the preparation of clinical nursing students will be appropriate for today's world.

The premise that guides this book is that every nursing faculty should prepare students to function in today's care environment, rather than preparing students for an envisioned "world of the future" or for a time when nursing care will be offered under ideal conditions. Failing to prepare students for the realities they will face does them no favor; nor does it serve to bring about a more desirable future. Indeed, only by preparing students to make an impact on the present world can we enable the next generation of nurses to participate in the creation of future health care environments.

Faculty members need not prefer the present system of managed care, but their teaching should prepare the student to cope with today's reality. In order for that to happen, they must understand the values and principles underlying the extant system. Today's system, confusing and constantly changing as it is, is dominated by managed care, a delivery system that has radically changed the roles of practicing nurses as well as other health care professionals, insurers, and even of patients and clients within the system. This book is not a primer on managed care, but a reflection on how the existence of that system should or might alter one's teaching in preparing students of nursing for their work in today's world.

1

The Managed Care Environment

To prepare students for today's health care environment, nursing faculty members must understand managed care, including the values that underlie delivery systems and the philosophy on which today's delivery rests. Nationwide, the health care industry has undergone a period of radical change resulting in a delivery system called *managed care*. Managed care is a series of strategies designed primarily to control and constrain costs for payers and, simultaneously, to preserve the quality of care. Managed care usually is initiated by insurers and employers to attain better health care for their dollar, in light of the increasing cost of health care. Mullahy (1995) offers the following definition:

> Managed care consists of the systems and mechanisms utilized to control, direct, and approve access to the wide range of services and costs within the health care delivery system. (p. 5)

> Managed care incorporates health maintenance organizations (HMOs), preferred provider organizations (PPOs), direct contracting (in which an employer contracts directly with a hospital or other health care facility), bill audits, utilization review, preadmission authorization, concurrent review, retrospective review, second surgical opinions (SSOs), independent medical exams (IMEs), and case management. (p. 5)

Flarey and Blancett (1996) describe managed care more simply, as an integrated delivery system that unites financing groups (insurers, employers) with providers, including hospitals, clinics, and physicians, home care, long-term-care facilities, and pharmacies. They see this organization as fast becoming the predominant infrastructure of our health care system (p. 3).

Managed care has numerous objectives, including but not limited to these: (1) less costly health care for those whose care is being managed, (2) fewer

1

episodes of illness, (3) shorter recuperative periods for clients, and (4) achievement of predetermined health care goals for clients. Although the clinical goals have always been important, the added objective is the fiscal constraint that allows purchasers and suppliers to hold down health care costs.

Because managed care is in part a set of strategies to control costs, it can be used in diverse settings. Often a managed care strategy is used in a traditional care facility; many acute care nursing services, for example, have adapted managed care strategies, including the use of case managers. Other managed care plans are put into place by insurers or employers. These plans may include case managers who oversee insurance reimbursements, or even case managers who develop health education programs in the workplace.

Although all managed care plans share the objective of reducing costs, they may look quite different because of their diverse settings. An employer's plan, for example, might include elements of what used to be called occupational health—with health education, routine exercise programs, weight and stress reduction, smoking cessation, and other health maintenance programs in the workplace. A plan put into place by an insurer might have aspects that look like public health nursing—with case finding and monitoring, especially for subscribers who have any condition known to be costly when it becomes acute.

Although different settings use different strategies, all share the characteristic that in deciding or recommending what will be done they interpose a third party between the health care provider and the patient. Decisions are reached or ratified only after considering aspects such as prevention, lifetime needs, desired outcomes for the patient, and total costs.

SOCIETAL REORGANIZATIONS OF HEALTH CARE

Any society, through its governmental systems, makes decisions concerning what aspects of life will be valued and how those values and their related products and activities will be distributed among its citizens. Health is one value among many—such as the arts, education, or leisure time. With rare exceptions, every society works in an environment of scarcity—that is, without the capability to implement all desirable goals. One convenient measure of a society's wealth is its gross domestic product (GDP), an index of the total market value of all the goods and services produced by a nation in a specified time period. Data on GDPs allow for international comparisons, as well as for determining the relative percentage of the GDP accounted for by any particular good or service—in our case, health care.

For a long time, the cost of health care rose proportionately faster and consumed a greater percentage of the GDP in the United States than that in

many other countries. In the United States, when health care costs continued to increase exponentially in the last two decades (finally approaching
14 percent of the GDP), concern was translated into action. The health care
industry voluntarily undertook measures to contain costs. But these early
efforts had only a minimal effect on slowing the accelerating costs of health
care. Part of the reason for the failure was that the health care industry
could not contain the rising costs of suppliers and other industries with
which it interacted.

The causes of increasing costs were easy to identify: developing technology, higher salaries for workers in the health care industry, rising cost of
equipment and supplies, and uncontrolled spending for each patient, with
no consideration of cost incurred. Any test or procedure that had the
potential to improve the patient's health, or the physician's knowledge of
the case, was used without reference to its cost. This was possible because
remuneration from insurers was based on costs incurred—what is today
called an *indemnity policy.*

Advancing medical technology had an indirect effect on health care
costs by enabling large numbers of people to live longer; and a new statistical group, the older old, required more medical monitoring and long periods of care in health facilities. Further, more and more extreme measures
were used with all critically ill patients in an attempt to prevent or delay
death, causing costly major resources to be consumed in the last days of
life for many patients. The problem of cost was further exacerbated by the
growing number of AIDS patients and by increasing lifestyle disorders
brought on by addiction and substance abuse.

The price of health insurance rose so fast that many small businesses
had difficulty remaining solvent when they provided coverage for employees. Many observers predicted that the social security health fund, the
national funding for Medicare and Medicaid, could soon become insolvent. Accurate or not, this projection rapidly brought about a change in the
federal reimbursement process. Providers of care for Medicare patients
would now be reimbursed through a "prospective payment system" that
tightly controlled costs, receiving a *per case payment* rather than reimbursement for costs incurred. Organizations would have to find frugal ways to
recover costs. Of course, those that instituted cost-effective management
could keep any unused funds if they managed to give care at less than the
reimbursed fee.

The system of *diagnosis-related groups* (DRGs) entered the scene as the
basis for setting prospective payment rates. DRGs were sets of patient
diagnoses clumped together, not on the basis of the clinical phenomena, but
on the basis of their use of resources. If items grouped together used approximately the same institutional resources (equipment; supplies; time of nurses,
physicians, and other care deliverers), then it could be assumed that they

cost approximately the same amount to deliver. Reimbursements would be based on the primary and secondary discharge diagnoses, not on the amount or type of care given in an individual case.

This change in reimbursement would make institutions develop systems to identify actual resources used by every patient. It became important to institutions to determine *outliers*, patients who ended up using more resources than predicted. Excessive use of resources could be traced to many different contributing factors, including the fact that patients with multiple health care problems might take longer to recuperate, and the fact that certain physicians might follow practice patterns requiring more intensive care.

One of the most accurate predictors of resource utilization, not surprisingly, was length of stay (LOS): the duration of a patient's stay in a care facility. All institutions providing acute and step-down care quickly learned that it paid to discharge patients as soon as possible. A fast turnover of patients became the best way for an institution to save money. Utilization of resources was also important. Overnight, conserving supplies and restricting unneeded tests became the rule. Cost of workers also became a factor; higher-paid workers could no longer be used for tasks that could be done by lower-paid workers.

Inevitably, imposition of the DRG system was the beginning of the system we now call managed care. The DRGs, with their prospective but controlled reimbursements, caused all institutions to reanalyze their health care delivery systems and structures. The system effectively enforced cost reduction, even at the expense of other values.

Few health care institutions could survive if their access to federal reimbursement programs was cut off, so virtually all were forced to adapt to the DRG reimbursement system. Soon other insurers also began adopting prospective payment programs. Health maintenance organizations (HMOs), which had preceded DRGs—a point worth emphasizing—were already using a prospective approach. The growth of these organizations was assured under managed care.

An HMO is a care delivery system based on a subscriber group of clients who receive all or a determined portion of their health care through the system. Its client fees were established without regard to the specific care given to any client. In essence, the HMO bases its financial calculations on *enrolled lives* rather than on what happens to specific clients. This system, called *capitation*, calculates cumulative prospective costs for a total group of clients, just as the DRG system calculated prospective costs per average case in a DRG category. Hence the DRG system and the HMO system established a new mind-set: prospective calculations based on predicted norms of usage. The system of regarding patients statistically, as groups rather than as individuals, had been established. The United States's failure to pass any form of universal health care plan has not basically altered the inevitable growth of managed care.

The slogans concerning health care under managed care usually concern two values seen as fulfilled simultaneously in the system: cost control and quality of care. Yet these two values clearly could be antithetical if unbalanced. For example, if patients are dismissed from care too early, without achieving the necessary health-related objectives, cost savings might be improved in the short run. However, in the long run this could incur greater costs as unattained but necessary health-related demands reasserted themselves. The issue becomes balancing these two goals, with an understanding that both must be achieved simultaneously.

In order to balance quality of care against cost, quality has to be assessed in some clearly definable way. Throughout the nation, the format became establishing *desired patient outcome goals* for each health condition or therapy. Achievement of the identified outcomes became the measure of quality. Chapter 3 will detail how such desired health care outcomes came to be elaborated in *clinical pathways*. Just as costs were calculated in the aggregate, clinical pathways were applied to patient groups, to a great extent supplanting the old system of having an individualized nursing care plan and medical plan for every patient.

The managed care system imposed a business mentality on health care providers, with bottom-line solvency the driving force in decisions. Whether it was a cause, an effect, or both, the DRG system accentuated the trend toward industrializing health care that was to emerge as managed care. Even if the specific DRG system itself is replaced in the future, the notion of controlled prospective payment has solidly taken hold in most reimbursement plans. It is highly unlikely that there will be any return to the old system of payment for costs incurred.

PREPAID ARRANGEMENTS AND MANAGED CARE PLANS

With the passage of the Health Maintenance Organization Act in 1973, other opportunities became available for prepaid plans, signaling a shift of medical care delivery to corporate arrangements and introducing new organizing formats into the health care environment. For all these plans, the notion was that, through planning, health care could be delivered more efficiently, more frugally, and with no loss in desired health outcomes. The system quickly revolutionized the health care environment. As Cohen and Cesta (1997) said:

> Managed care emerged as control shifted from the provider to the purchaser of health services. The managed care system links the provider with the

patient to manage cost, access, and quality components of the health care delivery. Major health policies like the federal Health Maintenance Organization Act, adopted in the early 1970s, established a trend for the growth of managed care programs. The HMOs and preferred provider organizations (PPOs), two popular examples, offered an alternative to costly inpatient care through the provision of cost-effective treatments and multiple preventive and outpatient services. (p. 32)

Today, there is extensive variation in managed health care plans, but several basic organizational structures are typical. The most common form is the health maintenance organization (HMO), which delivers health services—providing the financing and enrolling a population—for a fixed prepaid fee. The HMO group provides set benefits (often comprehensive) for enrolled members for a fixed dollar amount per time period per member. The industry speaks in terms of *paid lives.* Health maintenance organizations may have different sorts of providers, from physicians, chiropodists, and nutritionists to physical therapists. Some plans, like Oxford, admit nurse practitioners as members.

The HMOs relate to their providers in diverse ways, from the staff model to the independent practice arrangement to a network model. The *staff model* is the simplest arrangement. In this pattern, the health care providers are employees of the HMO, salaried workers who limit their practice to one employer, the HMO.

In the *independent or individual practice association (IPA) model,* a group of providers who are in practice for themselves join to form an association offering a full (or selected) spectrum of services to an HMO. The necessary peer review and utilization review are done by the health maintenance organization. Most IPAs take capitated payments from the HMO; others negotiate a mixed capitation and fee-for-service arrangement. Capitation is a method of payment for health services in which the provider (an individual or a group) is paid a fixed amount, calculated per covered life (by the number of members enrolled in the HMO), without regard to the actual services provided to the members.

An IPA provides an opportunity for physicians and other providers to remain in individual practices and work simultaneously with health maintenance organizations. A provider may have agreements with more than one HMO at the same time.

In the *network model,* an HMO contracts with two or more independent physician or provider groups. This is essentially a more complex form of the IPA model and is typical of the larger HMOs, many of which are national in size. In either of these forms, IPA or network, the HMO typically pays the contract group by capitation, per member per month (PMPM), with the contracting providers determining how those fees are split within their own group.

Other variations in HMO-provider arrangements deal with incentives designed to induce enrollees to choose one group of providers over others. In the *preferred provider organization (PPO) model,* the HMO selects as members certain health care providers (physicians and others) and directs its clients to these providers. Lists of providers are provided, referrals are kept within the group, and enrollees often get fuller reimbursements if they stay within the preferred provider network. Typically, the PPO offers the HMO a reduced cost (discounted capitation rate) in order to acquire the guaranteed patient population.

In the *exclusive provider organizations (EPO) model,* the EPO becomes the exclusive provider of care. (This is a more limited notion than the preferred provider organization.) Participants do not receive coverage for care provided by out-of-plan professionals. Developing an exclusive provider situation means that even more discounted rates may be negotiated between the HMO and the provider group, again because of guaranteed volume of business.

Not all physicians or other providers are content to negotiate with established HMOs. Many, instead, are becoming owners of their own capitation plans. In the past an employer group might pay an HMO, say, $150 per member per month. The HMO then might contract with a physician or provider group to deliver services at $120 per member per month. With this scheme, the HMO kept $30 per member risk-free, and the physician group was at risk of financial loss if more clients than anticipated needed care. Now many providers (primarily, though not exclusively physicians) are starting their own managed care organizations and negotiating directly with employers, avoiding the HMO middleman. Obviously such a plan needs up-front financing to start, but there is a developing pattern of increased provider-owned corporations.

Hospitals and other health care agencies are reimbursed through numerous methods under the new managed care systems, and not all managed care systems are derived from HMOs. Historically, in the early phases of managed care, a discount-off-charges was common. A per diem rate is also common today. In this arrangement, HMOs and PPOs are payed a fixed rate per day per patient, regardless of the amount of equipment or supplies, the number of procedures, or the use of ancillary services. In a per case or per stay reimbursement system, reimbursement is provided as a fixed sum regardless of the length of stay. The DRG system of payment typifies this arrangement.

Capitation arrangements use a different basis, paying the care agency a fixed amount per enrolled life per month whether or not the member uses the institution's services. In this arrangement, a care agency reaps more financial rewards if fewer enrollees use its facility or services.

Hence a hospital, for instance, can make money in the system even though it is not an HMO, provided that it negotiates advantageous managed care payment schemes. For example, if the number of patients actually admitted for care is less than the per capita rate negotiated, the financial edge will be in favor of the hospital. Similarly, if a patient on a per case reimbursement scheme is brought to a state of discharge rapidly (within a favorable length of stay), the hospital will be on the positive side fiscally. For the patient, of course, it is also desirable to recuperate faster, so everyone wins with a reduced length of stay if the health care goals are achieved.

Different payment schemes exist side by side at present, and different financial rewards are realized by the agency depending on the nature of the cases handled. From an institution's perspective, discount-off-charges and per diem contracting encourage longer stays to create a positive financial margin. In contrast, in payment on a per case basis, shorter stays and reduced consumption of resources lead to greater profit margins. In a capitated system, low facility usage means greater financial gain. While the payment schemes are still somewhat mixed, in general organizations profit more by decreasing patients' LOS. In other words, capitation and per case reimbursement plans predominate. From the perspective of the managed care plan, the key to solvency is effective actuarial planning and advantageous negotiation of contracts in a competitive market.

As a process, managed care develops over time within each geographic area. The development may take place in varying numbers of stages but Coile (1997) and Flarey and Blancett (1996, pp. 338–342) rely on a four-stage model attributed to APM Inc. (1992). In this model the first stage, an unstructured environment of independent providers and HMOs, is supplanted by the second stage, a loose framework of increasing HMO penetration, price pressures felt by providers, and the formation of loose provider networks. In the third stage consolidation of HMOs and PPOs occurs, with extensive mergers of institutions and extensive formation of group practices. In the fourth and final stage, integrated systems of managed patient care predominate in the managed competition arena. Each stage moves the given environment closer to a systems-based integrated system. Because of the patterns of growth and change, states and even different sections of the same state may differ in the character and extent of managed care.

In one of the more recent trends, point-of-service (POS) managed care plans have evolved to combat consumers' discontent with having their choice of providers limited. These arrangements typically use a primary provider as a gatekeeper for the services of other providers, limiting inappropriate use of specialists. However, the enrollee has some freedom in selecting his or her own providers. Such plans can range from open access to requiring the client to pay higher copayments for choosing providers outside of the network.

Variations of managed care continue to develop. From the perspective of the managed care system, relations tend to become more and more complex, creating an extensive web of providers and rules for operating within the system. Among provider organizations, much growth takes place outside the acute care setting, including ambulatory care centers, outpatient surgicenters, emergency care centers, hospices, rehabilitation institutions, home care organizations, diagnostic centers, and substance abuse centers. Such providers may be freestanding or part of a chain of organizations.

A chain of health care organizations may use a horizontal pattern, with all organizations of the same type—all nursing homes, for example, or all hospitals, or all surgicenters. A vertical chain links different types of provider organizations, allowing an HMO to keep enrollees within its network, and thus enhancing corporate profits. For example, such a corporation could move a patient from one of its acute care hospitals to a corporation-owned skilled care facility to a nursing home, all within the same network. The growth of nonacute care reflects the fact that profits flow from keeping patients out of hospitals, yet within the same provider system. Some vertical chains include businesses that supply or in some way service the provider organizations; other vertical chains may be massive corporations that include organizations unrelated to health care.

Not only has the move toward bottom-line management in health care changed the structure of health care organizations; it has also changed the tactics and strategies of management. Financial expertise is essential in negotiating contracts, and miscalculations may create financial jeopardy or even spell the end of a managed care system or of a contracting provider. From the perspective of the provider, the popular capitated systems clearly reward reduced delivery of services and reduced LOS. However, at the same time, to make a profit each care facility must strive to keep its beds and services filled. Thus, health care institutions are all striving for simultaneous increased turnover and increased volume of business. This means that organizations compete for the consumer. Competition is an inherent component of the managed care environment.

Not only are more customers needed in the health care delivery organization, but in an environment of declining fiscal resources (lower reimbursement rates), care delivery resources must be used more effectively and economically. Hence there is a focus on productivity. Unfortunately, in a labor-intensive field such as health care, productivity often means making do with fewer workers.

While economics is the driving engine of managed care, the second objective—quality of care—is not lost. Indeed, more and more insurers are collecting data on the performance of physicians and other health care providers (often reported in terms of patient outcomes and costs). For example, the Cleveland Health Quality Choice Coalition has completed outcome measures for 60 DRGs in hospital facilities used by their members

(Martin, 1997, p. 567). Similar groups are beginning to make such data available to consumers and consumer groups. Internally, such data may be used to determine what providers will be selected for plan enrollees. An enrollee, for example, may be told at what hospitals and by which surgeons his or her coronary bypass surgery may be performed. The enlightened managed care system wants to get a client the best mix of cost-efficient care plus desired care outcomes.

Nor is the design of health insurance companies and business insurance simple these days. There are insurance companies, reinsurance companies, and indemnity providers as well as self-insured businesses. Not all employers make health plan arrangements directly with HMOs. More employers are using health program brokers known as health insurance purchasing cooperatives (HIPCs). These firms examine all possibilities and negotiate with various health plans for their clients and employees.

Some employers are electing to be self-insured. This entails both risks and potential benefits. Such firms escape some of the legal stipulations that govern other insurers, and they usually experience an initial reduction in costs. Because of their limited numbers of enrollees, however, these businesses run a risk of having their health care funds depleted by a few highly expensive cases. To combat this vulnerability some businesses carry stop-loss insurance coverage in which a so-called reinsurance firm guarantees that it will step in and cover health benefits in excess of a set dollar limit.

One also can categorize plans according to the company's direct involvement in the provision of care. Larger companies are likely to have in-house case management; others may contract with independent case management firms.

In addition to all these new schemes, some people still prefer to carry traditional indemnity health plans. Such insurance still functions primarily on a fee-for-service basis, and it tends to be very expensive—but this is a price some are willing to pay for full freedom of choice in selecting their physicians, their other providers, and their care.

SUMMARY

Members of a nursing faculty need not know all the details of the emerging system of managed care. Indeed, that is possible only if one follows developments on a day-to-day basis. However, faculty members need to understand how the system has affected the nature of care delivery in this nation. Principles and common problems with the system will be described in chapter 2.

Here, we can say that the new system is characterized by much greater regulation of providers than in the past, consideration of patients primarily as aggregate groups, a focus on containing costs, a goal of preserving quality of care, a focus on productivity, and provision of a system of checks and balances through more structured controls of patients and providers (individuals and organizations).

REFERENCES

APM Inc. (1992). University Hospital Consortium and APM Incorporated Management Consultants.

Cohen, E. L., & Cesta, T. G. (1997). *Nursing case management: From concept to evaluation* (2nd ed.). St. Louis: Mosby–Year Book

Coile, R. (1997, January 30). Presentation for Case Management's Expert User's Forum, San Francisco, CA.

Flarey, D. L., & Blancett, S. S. (Eds.). (1996). *Handbook of nursing case management: Health care delivery in a world of managed care.* Gaithersburg, MD: Aspen.

Martin, C. J. (1997, April). Markets, Medicare, and making do: Business strategies after national health care reform. *Journal of Health Politics, Policy and Law, 22*(2), 557–590.

Mullahy, C. M. (1995). *The case manager's handbook.* Gaithersburg, MD: Aspen.

TEST YOUR UNDERSTANDING

Multiple-Choice
Select the one *best* answer.

1. *What is the driving force behind the creation of the managed care system?*
   a. To allow providers to manage care outcomes more predictably.
   b. To prevent employers from becoming insolvent because of excessive costs of health care coverage for employees.
   c. To control rising health care costs in government entitlement programs (Medicare and Medicaid).
   d. To provide assistance to the great number of uninsured people.

2. *Which of the following characteristics does* not *describe managed care?*
   a. Placing an intermediary between patient and provider.
   b. Paying a care facility only for services rendered.
   c. Setting predetermined goals for the outcome of care.
   d. Controlling to some extent the providers that an enrollee may use.

3. *What was the* chief *characteristic of the DRG-based plan for reimbursement? Reimbursement:*
   a. By case, not by care given.
   b. Given after the fact for care delivered.
   c. Covering only direct care given, with no additions for administrative costs.
   d. Covering only federal programs, not plans by private insurers.

4. *What is the logical connection between the two goals of reducing costs and improving quality of care?*
   a. Inverse relationship in the short term, but should covary over the long term.
   b. Direct relationship, where improving one is likely to improve the other.
   c. No relationship; they may be achieved independently of each other.

5. *In what way is the HMO managed care system like its predecessor, the DRG reimbursement system? Both:*
   a. Tend to pay less than the actual cost of caring for a patient.
   b. Pay prospectively.
   c. Are indemnity plans.

6. *How is payment made to a provider in a capitation plan? Payment depends on:*
   a. Number of enrollees cared for.
   b. Services rendered.
   c. Total number of enrollees in a plan.

Discussion of Answers

1. a. Care outcomes were important, but they did not give impetus to the creation of a new care delivery system.
   b. Many small employers were faced with serious threats to their existence because of rapidly expanding costs of employees' health care, but that was not the most powerful driving force.
   c. This is the correct answer.
   d. This problem remains even with managed care. It is as yet unaddressed in the laws of the United States.

2. a. The case manager makes major decisions, concerning what provider services will be reimbursed or what care procedures should be used. Hence, there is an intermediary between patient and provider.
   b. This is the correct answer.
   c. Most managed care programs have preset care outcomes that must be the goals of the providers.
   d. Most managed care programs control the choice of providers, for example through PPOs and EPOs.

3. a. This is the correct answer.
   b. This is false; reimbursement was given prospectively.
   c. Reimbursement was per case, not for actual direct care given.
   d. Reimbursement was quickly extended to private insurers as well.

4. a. This is the correct answer.
   b. Because better care is likely to cost more than less effective care, this relationship is wrong.
   c. As long as better care is likely to cost more rather than less, there is a relationship between these objectives.

5. a. Whether the paid fees are more or less than the actual cost depends on many variables, not simply whether it is a DRG or HMO system.
   b. This is the correct answer.
   c. Neither is an indemnity plan—that is, neither relates to actual costs.

6. a. Payment has nothing to do with the number of patients cared for.
   b. Payment has nothing to do with services rendered.
   c. This is the correct answer.

2

Problems and Promise in Managed Care

Many faculty members are predisposed to dislike the system of managed care, primarily because it may be incompatible with their preference for teaching the student to do "everything" for his or her assigned patients. In truth, there are both weaknesses and advantages to the managed care system. Both the good and the bad points, however, have implications for teaching nursing students. This chapter will identify some of the more common problems and promises.

PROBLEMS IN MANAGED CARE

Not everyone in the care delivery system is pleased with managed care. Not only is it a very complex system to operate, but there are other common complaints, including (1) the perceived dominance of cost control over quality of care (including reduction in the use of nurse professionals), (2) the interposing of a third party between patient and provider, and (3) the imperfect fit of the market supply-demand model.

Dominance of Cost Control Over Quality of Care

Chief among the complaints about managed care is the claim that costs are reduced by lowering the quality of care. In reviewing this criticism, as well as others that will follow, one must always differentiate between errors inherent in the system and errors that occur in the shakedown period when a system is evolving and being put in place. For example, early in the implementation of managed care, many enrollees found themselves switching providers at the behest of their new plans. Clearly, the game of musical chairs played among clients and providers was costly both economically and in terms of quality of care. Patients were forced to give up providers who were intimately acquainted with their health needs and to take on providers who would have to learn their needs. The system fractured long-standing client-provider relationships, many of which would never be replaced in kind. Such a system in no way favors cost savings or quality control in the short run. Yet this game of musical chairs was a start-up situation rather than one that was to dominate an in-place system.

One hopes that many of the complaints of decreased quality of care may be attributed to start-up phenomena. However, it is clear that there are potential conflicts between the two principles of reducing costs and improving or maintaining quality of care. Many managed care programs claim that to some degree, care can be made more efficient and streamlined without loss of quality. This is true, but there comes a point when efficiency has been optimized, and further cost saving will have an impact on quality of care.

Quality of care can be defined many ways, including but not limited to these: (1) the achievement of appropriately selected patient outcomes; (2) patients' and families' satisfaction with care over the time it was received; (3) prompt identification of and remedies for negative side effects; (4) relief of pain, discomfort, and anxiety; (5) patients' sense that they are in good hands, that is, they have appropriate stewardship; (6) appropriate measures to enhance recuperation and long-term fitness; and (7) that all the above are received in a timely fashion. To repeat: these definitions are not exhaustive; they are offered to suggest the comprehensive definition of quality of care. Nevertheless, in keeping with the common practice in managed care, we will use the term *quality of care* to mean the achievement of desired, predetermined patient outcomes. The other measures are important, but they may be more difficult to quantify for system tracking.

Several factors have been identified as affecting quality of care under managed care plans. One factor is the decreased use of professionals, with unlicensed personnel doing tasks once assigned to RNs, with nurse practitioners doing tasks previously assigned to interns and even residents, and with providers of all sorts being penalized if their practice is "overzealous" in the use of tests, equipment, or inpatient days. It is true that some plans remove from their roster of providers those physicians whose practice is more costly than the norm. All these moves save on costs; but on the face of it, one cannot assert that quality will always be unaffected.

Another factor affecting quality is the mistaken early discharge of patients as a way to reduce costs. Are patients being sent home or to step-down care too soon? There are certainly enough stories to let us know that this occasionally happens. The issue is whether these incidents are mistakes in judgment or are systematically fostered by a plan that puts cost savings above quality of care.

All this is not to say that the most expensive care—namely, acute care—is always the best. For example, a patient who is ready for a different and "lower" level of care may benefit greatly from being placed in step-down care in the community. A more expensive acute care facility often is not prepared to deal with necessary rehabilitation procedures. Patients' learning, to take another example, is often better achieved in step-down care than in the hectic acute care facility. Each care setting has its strengths and limitations, and the managed care environment should place the patient in the right setting at the right time.

Many people propose that the system favored cost over quality at its inception, but that it is now being brought back into line. Whatever the facts of the case, professionals must be on guard to see that professional standards are not disregarded, and this calls for courage if the system is rigid or slow in responding to providers' input. Clearly, there is potential tension between the two extremes of the pendulum, cost and quality, if the concepts are misapplied.

EDUCATIONAL IMPLICATIONS

Faculty members must assume there will be greatly enhanced use of nurse helpers—technicians as well as minimally trained personnel. Student nurses at all levels will need to learn how to manage subordinate personnel effectively, including how to evaluate and supervise their work. In this respect, the managed care system is more complex than its predecessor, and it requires more advanced managerial skills, even from a beginning nurse. Faculty members who were previously immersed in the primary care model of one-to-one care will need to modify their exclusive focus on clinical nursing. It is no longer enough for nurses to learn one-to-one care, nurse-to-patient. They must also learn nurse-to-nurse management, that is, supervising others providing care. This works two ways: it may involve supervising (1) lower-level unlicensed personnel or (2) personnel with more education than the nurse or student nurse. For example, students may find a clinical specialist on their assigned team.

In order to fulfill a managerial role, even basic students must learn techniques of supervision, delegation, and evaluation of personnel, as well as how to determine the capacities of others to perform such tasks. Capacities will have to be judged on individual, institutional, and legal grounds: (1) What is the performance capability of the individual? (2) What performances (task and responsibilities) are to be assigned according to institutional job descriptions? (3) What tasks can a given level of personnel perform within the nursing and medical practice acts of the state?

In addition to looking at the performance of tasks and qualifications (who can do what), today's student needs a focus on achieving patient outcomes. An orientation to specific tasks is not enough. The patient outcome that results from each task is the central theme. For example, instead of teaching a student the "right way" to do a given procedure, the teacher might explore several methods, considering which would achieve the desired patient outcome most efficiently in a given situation. The focus on outcomes is crucial to both performance and supervision in a managed care environment.

Interposing a Third Party Between Patient and Provider

Among the common criticisms leveled at managed care is the loss of clinical autonomy by the health care practitioner. This occurs because managed care organizations often require case managers to make clinical judgments based on protocols that may not consider differences among individual patients. This practice puts pressure on physicians or nurses who vary from the normative procedures. Managed care programs attempt to direct providers' behavior, using both the stick and the carrot—they are controlled or incentivized, as Morreim (1997, p. 334) says. The carrot may include such aspects as financial incentives for primary providers (e.g., bonuses and capitation gains for cost-effective practice; p. 333). The stick may include "deselecting" physicians whose practice patterns do not fit with the organization's preferences (p. 334). Indeed, there are physicians threatening lawsuits over such deselection, claiming "restraint of trade."

Additionally, some prominent physicians (those who can rely on drawing a clientele apart from the reimbursement plans) are electing to withdraw from HMO and managed care plans that severely limit their practice preferences, as well as those whose capitation plans or fees for patient visits are judged too low.

Morreim notes (as others have noted) that the "carrot" financial incentives for the physician may arouse the patients' distrust and cause them to suspect that a physician puts his or her own interest first. Morreim also notes that managed care plans may be particularly at odds with the academic health care center because plans are reluctant to cover the latest technologies and innovative treatments (p. 333), and these are major driving forces at an academic health center.

Nurses will find themselves on both sides of this issue of intervention by a third party. Nurse practitioners, for example, may react like physicians to controls placed on them by a managed care plan. On the other side, probably the majority of case managers—the interveners—are nurses, and this opens up a new range of interesting employment opportunities.

EDUCATIONAL IMPLICATIONS

For nursing faculty members, the task will be to make students understand that managed care protocols and directives guide but do not dictate the nature of their practice. Some level of autonomy may be sacrificed for the sake of standard operating procedures. If two methods are equally effective, the student may be directed to use the less costly one, for example. Students today must understand that the managed care system, along with its protocols, is based on numbers, patient norms, and universal standards. This is in contrast to the once prevailing nursing philosophy, which placed great emphasis on the patient as a unique individual.

The standard care protocol (often in the form of a clinical pathway) is both a blessing and a curse from the teacher's perspective. It provides a convenient, relatively safe crutch for an insecure student; but at the same time it may discourage independent thinking. Hence, a new balancing act must be taught—that is, the balancing of normative patient needs and programs of care against unique and individualized patient needs that exist despite normative care plans.

While learning to work within protocols and directives, the student (and the faculty member) must understand that such guidelines never remove nurses' ultimate responsibility for their own practice decisions. Nurses are expected (and required) to exercise their own judgment, even in the application of guidelines. This means that the nurse must know when a guideline becomes inapplicable in an individual case. When a client deviates from the outcomes anticipated, the nurse must assess, report, and deal with the relationship between process and outcome. The nurse should look for and expect variance; there is no such thing as functioning on autopilot.

Imperfect Fit of the Market Supply-Demand Model

Managed care is characterized by the fact that it introduces market principles into health care, putting economic considerations and competition into play. This means that the health care industry is subject to the same market ideology as are other businesses. Yet the industrial model of supply and demand is not a perfect fit in health care. As Martin (1997) notes, differences arise because of several factors:

> Third party insurers interrupt the natural balance between providers and patients or supply and demand. Health is (often literally) a life-and-death

issue where rational decision making is at its most problematic. As a society we are unwilling to forget about the sick patient who is unable to meet the costs of his or her amelioration. (p. 557–558)

Many issues of supply and demand have yet to be answered. Chief among them is the care available for the uninsured. Supply and demand are also creating three- and four-level tiers of health care, bringing into question concerns over whether health care is a right or a purchase that can be made for different qualities and levels of care. At the moment, older notions of health care as a right appear to be losing out to notions of health care as a purchase.

Another problem is how to deal with those who have "orphan" diseases or who are outliers on projected clinical pathways. People who don't fit into the norms or into aggregate diagnoses and behaviors create problems for the system and, secondarily, for themselves. A system based on norms is not ready to deal with market demands for an unusual product—for instance, research on cures for unusual diseases. A related problem is how those who already have a known, expensive health condition will be able to find insurance without having to impoverish themselves in order to qualify for help (if they qualify at all). Managed care plans have much to lose in admitting such persons as members. If problems such as these are handled entirely on market principles, many people will suffer from lack of medical care. Clearly, the system will require some intervention to alleviate the stresses created by a purely market-driven operation.

The negative interpretation of managed care is typified by Mechanic (1997), who notes community opposition to managed care as reflected in legislation and referenda that may or may not be wise. He sees health professionals and consumer groups using "atrocity incidents," particularly emotionally laden issues such as early discharge following childbirth and mastectomy, "gag rules" that prevent providers from discussing all options with clients, and physician incentives that undermine patients' beliefs in physicians as their agents (p. 181). Obviously, many of the things that are wrong with managed care have to do with a misalignment of incentives, and the system must work to change these errors.

THE PROMISE OF MANAGED CARE

Cost Control

Despite its problems, managed care has certain promise for the overall status of health care in the nation. First, it does have the potential to control the very real problem of runaway health care costs. Despite increased administrative costs within the system, it seems better able to respond to economic demands than the previous system of uncontrolled costs was. Clearly, the cost of the health care system cannot be allowed to escalate without any constraints. Clearly, also, voluntary constraints were not working in the old system. Managed care forces all parties (providers, payers, patients) to consider the price of health care. It oversees and controls the use of health care resources. True, controls on costs may need vigilant balancing and refinement, but it is hoped that the system will be able to take this factor into account. Further, managed care has forced health care providers to think in terms of aggregate populations in a manner previously reserved for public health providers. Clearly, the care of majority groups is where attention should be place in the case of scarce resources.

Focus on Outcomes

Additionally, managed care has proved itself strong in identifying standards for patient outcomes and in collecting data on outcomes. Having clearly defined goals and clinical pathways of care for various patient groups is a keystone for evaluating this system. Relating therapies to outcomes in the managed care system allows us truly to see what our health care dollars are purchasing.

Systems Orientation

Another distinct promise in managed care is the fact that it takes a systems orientation to heart. In the geographic sections of the country in the later stages of market evolution, full-spectrum integrated systems emerge. Large managed care systems weave together a conglomerate of health care delivery facilities and providers, creating a comprehensive delivery system. From the viewpoint of the patient, this is reflected in the primary physician, who oversees and coordinates any care by specialists. Hence, someone has a "view from the top," ensuring that the patient has a comprehensive group of specialists working in concert toward meeting his or her needs. Similarly, the case manager guides the patient through the coordinated system to the appropriate facilities and services.

Moreover, managed care is rapidly changing the settings in which care is delivered. Instead of a system focused on acute care, a health care system that utilizes multiple care settings is evolving. Despite the apparent logic of these placement selections, however, not all studies confirm cost savings at this stage of system development.

EDUCATIONAL IMPLICATIONS

The movement to multiple settings radically changes the teaching role, because students need to learn to function in different places, with diverse groups of clients—from the acute to the convalescent to those requiring health maintenance. Most faculty members feel that the movement to diverse settings is a good thing, for several reasons. First, it gives students experience in functioning in diverse settings. Second, it opens up many new opportunities for students' clinical experience if the local neighborhood is short of placements in acute care settings.

These advantages are not as simple as they appear. Using a diversity of settings greatly complicates teaching in that it adds a new element, *context*, to the learning requirements. The application of a single principle in diverse settings, with diverse populations, for example, is not something a student will understand on the basis of a context-free lecture or demonstration. For example, conservation of a patient's energy will appear radically different in moving from the acute care facility to home care. Students need to "relearn" content in every unique setting, even if the content was previously familiar. New content makes learning a double task. To assume that "general content" can be specifically applied in any context is an error made by inexperienced teachers.

Take, as illustration, our example of conservation of a patient's energy. In the acute care facility, the student is likely to think of this as a physiological principle to be assessed from the viewpoint of the patient's body. In home care for a recuperating factory worker, however, the focus might shift to sociological and economic considerations, requiring a different mind-set on the part of the student.

Nor is adaptation to new contexts the only challenge for teachers who are moving students out of a learning environment dominated by the acute care setting. In the extended settings, students must be challenged to function with independent (and sometimes isolated) autonomy, simply because these step-down settings may have fewer people available to consult. Worse, with the present economic cutbacks faced by schools of nursing, faculty members may also be in scarce supply at any given facility. In placement at nonacute settings, students are more likely to find themselves on their own. Because of this increased demand for independent functioning, nursing education must move toward a more active decision-making model of caregiving, as opposed to any notion of the nursing role as merely facilitative, supportive, or passive.

Additionally, learning must now involve how systems function and how one manages from inside a system. A systems orientation is essential if a student is to function in diverse settings within a care delivery system. However one views managed care, it has made the nursing role more complex, and this means that the faculty cannot merely teach the clinical content of nursing but must include in the students' education their role in the matrix of present-day care.

Focus on Quality Assurance

One of the greatest promises of managed care is the opportunity it presents for research into patient care. With clearly defined patient outcomes, as well as specified clinical pathways, the managed care system facilitates not only institutionwide but systemwide and multisystemwide quality assurance measurement. On the micro level, clinical pathways define goals for patient care against which outcomes may be compared. On the macro level, one such measurement tool (used on the managed care system level) is Health Plan Employer Data and Information Set (HEDIS). This is a widely used measure of performance that presently includes 75 measures, allowing comparisons among managed care systems. Additionally, the National Committee for Quality Assurance (NCQA) spearheads the effort to assess, measure, and report on the quality of care provided by managed care organizations. This independent organization has an accreditation process for HMOs.

The quality of health care is a consuming interest for everyone, and managed care creates systems that can be used to measure quality of care as well as cost. A common equation states that the value of health care is quality plus service, divided by the price.

GENERAL NURSING ISSUES

As a case manager and supervisor of other care personnel, the nurse is pushed to a level of accountability not seen in prior eras. When most nurses worked in acute care settings, difficult decisions could be referred to (or discussed with) a convenient group of peers. In contrast, many nurses in home care and step-down care now lack such a peer group. Independent decision making and professional autonomy are no longer matters of choice but are imposed on nurses in all settings, whether or not they are ready for this level of responsibility. Although protocols for care add an element of standard operating procedure, many new settings add a need for individual professional functioning and autonomous decision making. Even in acute care, it is no longer true that "a nurse is a nurse is a nurse." Effective nursing vice presidents can no longer afford to keep a nurse employee who is dependent and avoids making decisions.

In addition to demanding more independent decision making, the managed care system also forces the various health care professionals to work together, sharing patient care goals in ways that were not heard of a decade or more ago. Once, nursing isolated "nursing goals" for its patients and devoted its quality control measures to these goals. Now nurse professionals must cooperate with other professionals to achieve shared goals. Most clinical pathways, for example, assume an interface: several professionals may be working jointly toward the achievement of any given goal for a patient. This ideology calls for a major change in the nursing role: cooperation instead of competition, with mutual respect for other professionals, and making overt one's contributions to patient care.

EDUCATIONAL IMPLICATIONS

In the past, faculty members have focused on what makes nursing different from medicine, social work, or other professions. The outlook was insular and isolating. Now the faculty must focus instead on commonalities and shared vision among professionals. In the best teaching reorganizations, this involves shared classes or clinical experiences for students in all the various health professions.

This pattern is in distinct contrast with a faculty's focus on discrete nursing theories and unique nursing terminology—for example, making nursing diagnoses that were different from medical diagnoses. Nursing faculties now have to question this kind of insularity and seek ways to participate in greater intimacy with professional peers. This also calls for instilling a different philosophy of teamwork in nursing students, as well as finding ways for the diverse health professions to interact during the student years.

SUMMARY

Managed care has advantages and limitations for all those concerned. The nursing faculty member will need to convey these promising and problematic aspects to students who are to work in the system. Today's nurse will need to be more self-directed, more versatile, and better able to work effectively with others. To achieve this, the faculty will need to question long-held values and predispositions that have been passed along to nursing students in the past. The nursing role must be inculcated and taught as an active decision-making role. It is true that we give lip service to this model, but we often do so in ways that discourage nursing students from acting on their own decisions.

REFERENCES

Martin, C. J. (1997, April). Markets, Medicare, and making do: Business strategies after national health care reform. *Journal of Health Politics, Policy and Law, 22*(2), 557–590.

Mechanic, D. (1997, June 11). Managed care as a target of distrust. *Journal of the American Medical Association, 277*(22), 1810–1811.

Morreim, E. H. (1997, May). Managed care, ethics, and academic health centers: Maximizing potential, minimizing drawbacks. *Academic Medicine, 72*(5), 332–338.

TEST YOUR UNDERSTANDING

Multiple-Choice
Select the one *best* answer.

1. *The solution to which of the following problems has been advanced by the shift to managed care systems?*
   a. Developing good interpersonal relations between clients and providers.
   b. Making care decisions based on patient outcomes.
   c. Advancing research on new methods of care technology.

2. *How has managed care structured relations among and between the various health care professions?*
   a. It has decreased the need for interactions among health care professionals.
   b. It has made no difference in professional relationships in any way.
   c. It has increased the need for interactions among health care professionals.

3. *Which nursing value may be most challenged in the managed care system?*
   a. The need for a separate nursing diagnostic system.
   b. The need for professional autonomy and decision making.
   c. The need to streamline procedures and practices.

4. *Why might a person with an "orphan" (rare) disease be at a disadvantage in a managed care system?*
   a. The system is geared toward patients who fall within statistical norms.
   b. The system does not favor use of specialists who may be required for care of patients with orphan diseases.
   c. The orphan diseases require too much time in acute hospital care.

5. *Why did the legislature become involved in regulating the length of time new mothers and their infants could remain hospitalized?*
   a. There was too much diversity from one managed care plan to another.
   b. It perceived that managed care put cost above safe care.
   c. It was responding to hysterical, invalid public protest.

Disucssion of Answers

1. a. Managed care has placed physicians in positions where they profit for giving less comprehensive care. Patients are aware of this, and it has impaired good interpersonal relations.
    b. This is the correct answer.
    c. Managed care is based on doing things the least expensive way. Most such programs do not want to contribute to the cost of research and development of new techniques.

2. a. Clinical pathways often require professionals to work together toward shared goals.
    b. Interfaces between professionals have been affected in many ways. Competition, for example, may have pitted different professions against each other in seeking clients.
    c. This is the correct answer.

3. a. This is the correct answer.
    b. Despite standard protocols for much patient care, the nurse in the new system will need to demonstrate enhanced autonomy and decision making, for example in isolated settings where he or she may be the only nurse present.
    c. Streamlining of all processes is in keeping with attempts by managed care to achieve cost-effectiveness. This value is supported, not challenged.

4. a. This is the correct answer.
    b. The system controls specialist care but does not disfavor it when required.
    c. The orphan disease is disfavored not specifically because of the time spent in acute care, but because of many factors, including its long-range costs.

5. a. While there may have been some diversity among plans, that factor did not cause legislative interference.
    b. This is the correct answer.
    c. The public response was not unwarranted; serious life-threatening incidents have occurred.

3

Case Management

One component of managed care is case management: a system in which one person, the case manager, is made accountable for the achievement of planned health care outcomes for an individual patient or a client group. Case management is not a new concept; it has always been in effect in community health care, where nurses and social workers have traditionally carried a caseload of patients specifically assigned to them. Historically, case management has led to mergers and networking among institutions so as to achieve a focus on the client who is weaving among and between these various care delivery centers. Yet the concept has received new appreciation in the managed care system. Case management consists of overseeing, evaluating, and when necessary intervening in the planned care for an individual through the duration of an illness or through the duration of the person's time within a designated managed care system.

THE CASE MANAGER

The case manager, as Mullahy (1995) says, "is the catalyst who sifts through the array of possible paths, selects the most appropriate plan, and then coordinates the expertise and support of other professionals, family members, agencies, and suppliers" (p. 3). A case manager may be employed by a health care provider, a care delivery system, or a payer (an employer or insurer), or may work for an independent case management business.

Most case managers that members of a nursing faculty encounter will work in hospitals, home health agencies, and various step-down and rehabilitation units in the *provider* sector. In these settings, the case manager is usually a nurse or a social worker, although in some systems physicians may fill the role. The case manager is accountable for the patient's pattern of care and its outcome.

A case manager employed in the *payer* sector may work for an insurance carrier, a third-party administrating agency, an independent case management program, or one of various types of health maintenance organizations. The work role here, while it has the same goals as the role of a case manager in the provider sector, tends to be more administrative, less clinical, although clinical judgments will be involved. A case manager in the payer sector typically tracks all hospital admissions and other circumstances whereby the employing agency may incur costly reimbursements. These case managers often are thought of as mere claims managers, but ideally the role is much more. Case managers on the payer side, while often nurses or social workers, may also be people who have had experience administering workers' compensation and disability programs. If such managers lack specific medical knowledge, they are often teamed with a health care professional.

Case managers on the payer side typically focus on the 3 to 5% of patients who account for 60 to 70% of the expenditures (Mullahy, p. 6). The same may be true of case management programs under early development in health care delivery systems. While such systems tend to grow and eventually cover most patient cases, they usually begin with those cases likely to be most costly. Mullahy identified certain diagnoses—head injury, multiple trauma, cancer, AIDS, organ transplants, cardiovascular disease, stroke, burns, spinal cord injury, premature birth, and high-risk pregnancy— as falling within the "most costly" category (p. 6). Cohen and Cesta (1993), working on the provider side, identify those with AIDS and the elderly population (pp. 49–54). Whatever the high-cost groups are, they can be monitored with case management, and appropriate preventive measures can be taken to avoid or decrease the number of expensive acute episodes. Many systems also include education and motivational–behavior modification plans as essential parts of prevention, as well as ongoing monitoring.

In each case, the case manager aims to achieve the following objectives, albeit in different ways:

1. Allow for collaborative practice and planning among all health care professionals involved in a patient's case.
2. Coordinate providers and payers for an agreement on the best plan of care.
3. Define or follow protocols that identify desired client outcomes and therapeutics.
4. Focus on rapid and effective achievement of desired outcomes.
5. Prevent acute episodes through interventions.

6. Foster early discharge from health care facilities and programs.
7. Increase efficient use of health care resources.
8. Intervene in therapies of any and all providers that are ineffective in achieving set outcome goals in a timely and cost-effective manner.

One of the great advantages of case managers' serving on the payer side is that more reimbursement is typically allowed for prevention and rehabilitation. For example, under the old system of payment by indemnity coverage, a patient would never be reimbursed for such items as a special home toilet seat or an air filter. Yet payer-employed case managers know the value of such preventive reimbursements. Inexpensive reimbursements in health maintenance pay off fiscally as well as in patient outcomes. Continuing-care models of case management take the long view of health outcomes and cost for their clients.

CHANGES FOSTERING DEVELOPMENT OF CASE MANAGEMENT

Case management grew out of the goals of managed care: quality care and savings in costs. Quality of care can best be measured by the achievement of predetermined outcome goals, usually identified for groups of patients and thereafter modified as required for any given individual. As we said earlier, cost is closely related to length of stay for inpatient facilities; therefore, it makes sense to strive to achieve desired outcomes in the shortest possible time—a goal that should please the client as well as the provider. Controlling or preventing chronic conditions that would be expensive if they became acute is a tactic best handled through employer and payer case management.

OUTCOME MEASURES

In an inpatient facility, outcome standards are typically developed in *clinical pathways* (also called *critical paths* or *case maps*) for selected diagnoses, problems, or therapies. The clinical pathway describes a blended plan of care (constructed by all providers, considering the subject together) as well as a day-by-day schedule identifying when the elements of the plan will be enacted and the time by which each interim or final outcome goal should be achieved. Clinical pathways are set up in many different ways. Table 3.1 shows one such structure. Refer to Flarey and Blancett (1996) and Blancett and Flarey (1996) for extensive examples of clinical pathways.

Clinical pathways provide a guide against which the case manager can compare the progress of each patient. If a patient fails to progress on

TABLE 3.1   Sample Format for a Clinical Pathway

Patient: Diagnosis: Projected length of stay:		Unit: DRG:		
Terminal outcome desired:				
Day 1 Intermediate goal	Procedures	Physician:	Variation	Corrective action
		Nurse:		
		Nutritionist:		
		Physical therapist:		
Day 2 (continues as day 1)				

schedule, the manager can consult with the provider or providers account-able for the mediating therapies in order to modify the plan. Payer and HMO case managers may use similar clinical pathways for clients with chronic diseases.

Like the rest of managed care, the strategy of case management reflects a new way of thinking about health care delivery, moving us from a per-spective that views each individual patient as highly unique, and thus focuses on the qualitative issues of care, to a viewpoint that sees most patients as somewhat alike. The use of clinical pathways, for example, assumes that large numbers of patients can be treated in a similar fashion.

This quantitative, normative, group orientation brings together issues of quality and a quantitative viewpoint. This is one of the chief changes brought about in today's managed care: a shift from an individualized orientation focused on quality to an group orientation focused on quality plus quantity.

FORMS OF CASE MANAGEMENT

Managed care, as noted in Chapter 1, is a collection of strategies used by insurers and providers to influence health care decisions. It helps clients know when they need care, helps them get that care, and controls the care. Within that context, case management is used in diverse settings.

Even institutions that do not have a mandate to apply case management often do so. Many hospitals, for example, use it as a strategy to control their own costs. Providers' movement toward case management, borrowing from community health, has spread to acute care facilities and then out to other inpatient facilities. Often the first step in case management is creating the clinical pathways that guide a case manager. A given pathway is created by having all the concerned professionals work together.

Case management takes place under many structural arrangements, including these:

1. Separate business selling case management services.
2. Subsidiary of a company whose business is not health but which wants case management for its employees.
3. Subsidiary or department of an insurance company.
4. Subsidiary of a health care organization that manages total patient care—HMOs and PPOs are examples.
5. Separate department in an acute care hospital or another health care facility.
6. Separate department within a nursing division.
7. Decentralized function that is assigned to various departments of a nursing division.
8. Function performed on various nursing units with one or more assigned case managers.
9. Assignment for a bedside nurse who is expected to perform case management functions along with her care role (Barnum & Kerfoot, 1995, p. 89).

Case management has grown as a response by payers to expensive health care. Companies such as American Telephone and Telegraph and Chrysler, as well as insurers such as Kaiser Permanente, employ case managers for employees and policyholders who account for a substantial portion of the health services given or reimbursed.

The organizational arrangements for case management vary, depending on the circumstance. For example, insurance companies and business and industrial employers hire case managers to oversee their enrollees or employees, as do private case management firms. Acute care hospitals often use case managers for all admitted patients, regardless of their insurance or managed care plans. The hospital setting is probably the one most likely to be of importance to faculty members, because it is here that students will be likely to interface with case managers and clinical pathway protocols.

CLINICAL PATHWAYS

A clinical pathway is a protocol of care developed for a group of patients who share a diagnosis, treatment plan, or problem. The plan, typically covering care delivered by all professionals, is used as a directive for care and as a set of criteria for evaluating ongoing care. These clinical pathways are made up of protocols developed like GANTT charts, which display a total project step by step, indicating when each element will be initiated, carried out, or stopped. Hence, each day of an illness or of care for a given condition (or therapy/surgery) is marked with key events of care and expected levels of recuperation. Patients are expected to stay "on course"; otherwise, the case manager will discuss the variances with the professional or professionals seen as influencing the outcome. Variances in projected therapies, especially those that are more costly than the norm, will be discussed with the appropriate professional.

While it is not necessary to have clinical pathways in order to implement case management, this is the common procedure. In managed care systems, clinical pathways usually are developed by panels of experts. In provider institutions, recovery trajectories are determined by the various professionals working together or are purchased commercially and modified for the given institution. Nursing, medicine, and social work are usually involved in codetermining clinical pathways.

Under the leadership of a director of case management, each participant defines the current practices of his or her profession and examines the desired outcomes and practices leading to them. Outcomes will vary from institution to institution and from community to community, in light of local standards of practice. The identified patient outcomes become part of the case management protocol. Where necessary, clinical pathways can be modified for particular patients, but the normative patterns guide management of most cases. As noted above, the case manager ensures that the patient stays on the path as the case progresses or else seeks explanations for variances from the pattern.

Thus, the case manager continuously monitors assigned patients for variances from their plotted recuperation trajectories. When a variance occurs, the case manager seeks out the causes, discusses it with the appropriate professionals, seeks solutions to obstacles, and alters the plan of care so as to achieve the desired outcomes. However the details of the clinical pathway are displayed, they tell who should do what, correlating everyone and everything with the patient's interim outcomes and final desired outcomes.

In terms of research and evaluation, there is an obvious advantage to handling a large number of patients on the same clinical pathway. Such a system allows for easy application of research designs. Subsequent modifications in protocols, again for large numbers of patients, can quickly associate changes in protocols with changes in patient outcomes.

MODELS OF CASE MANAGEMENT

Many different forms of case management may be seen in an acute care facility where faculty members are often involved with students. In this setting, it is common to employ nurses as case managers. Sometimes a single nurse fills the roles of both primary nurse and case manager simultaneously. Such a person is responsible for patient care from admission to discharge (or later), with emphasis on length of stay (LOS); for writing the nursing care orders; and for delegating care to associates when he or she cannot deliver it (or on off-shifts). This model has the advantage of using assignment patterns closest to those already in effect in many acute care facilities. A limitation of the model, however, is that the orientation toward case management may be lost if the nurse becomes immersed in primary care functions.

More often, the case manager is a nurse or social worker with a caseload, determined either by type of patient case (so that cases may be distributed over several units) or by the physical placement of patients on in-house units. A typical unit using the latter design might have three or four case managers. In these designs, the case manager reviews cases, discussing them with head nurses or with primary care nurses and assigned caretakers. The case manager also discusses the plan and its achievement with nonnurse professionals involved in the patient's care (physicians, social workers, nutritionists, physiotherapists, and others). In these cases, case managers function like their counterparts in the payer sector, with more emphasis on planning and controlling, and less emphasis on actual care delivery. As with the direct care model, the case manager in this in-house design is responsible for a patient's care and related outcomes throughout the entire episode of illness, no matter who delivers the actual care.

In an acute care setting, the case manager will need access to much information, including information related to DRGs, costs, allotted LOS, outliers, and the procedures attached to each DRG. The manager must also have access to information about the case mix index, the cost of resources, and resource consumption (Tahan, 1993, pp. 54–55).

Because the whole managed care system relies on norms, variance analysis becomes an important function of the case manager. The first concern is budget variances and patients' variances from critical pathways and projected LOS. Operational variances can also occur, that is, delays in care applications because of failures in the institutional operations systems. For example, surgery may be delayed because of scheduling complications, or a plan to move a patient to a long-term-care bed may be delayed because of communications errors.

Faculty members need to sensitize students to variations in case management plans and to how any given plan is integrated into the operations of the care facility. Whatever the role for which the students are being prepared, they should be able to identify how that role interfaces with the relevant case management roles.

IMPLEMENTING A CASE MANAGEMENT SYSTEM

Implementing a case management system requires a clear administrative plan, including job descriptions for case managers, stating their accountability and authority, as well as clear identification of how the managers interface with others in the system. The powers of case managers are critical if they are to negotiate with other professionals. The role will be quite different, for example, for a case manager who is a "modified" head nurse in an acute care facility and a case manager who is making reimbursement decisions in an insurance company.

Gaining the acceptance of providers can be difficult in any setting, because most providers are resistant to having an intermediary make judgments concerning their care. The system, designed to keep costs at a minimum, has been known to cause such resistance that some providers (particularly physicians) may withdraw from managed care programs rather than comply with the interventions. Other caregivers, though, recognize the advantage of case management and are pleased when more efficient and effective alternatives are offered for care interventions.

For the consumers, the system, with its checks and balances, may require more "bookwork," such as arranging for approved referrals from their plan's primary physicians. Yet many consumers see a lower cost, such as the minimal copayments or no copayments featured in many plans. Consumers' satisfaction is improved if there are clear directives from the case managers. Most large managed care systems, for example, have well established communication systems and 24-hour lines for consumers' queries.

Tahan (1996) elaborates a ten-step process for developing case management plans in an acute care system: (1) designing the format of the plan, (2) selecting the target population, (3) organizing an interdisciplinary team, (4) educating the team about the process, (5) examining current practice, (6) reviewing the literature, (7) determining the length of the plan, (8) writing the content, (9) conducting a pilot study, and (10) standardizing the plan (pp. 113-120).

EDUCATIONAL IMPLICATIONS

Some graduate programs are specifically designed to prepare nursing case managers, but those curricula are not the subject of this chapter. Instead, we look at how the existence of case managers should affect the teaching of nursing students. Clearly, students will need to know the role and functions of case managers who operate in the clinical sites where they practice. Typically, case managers work within a matrix with head nurses (with whatever title they have). The head nurse has "geographic" and organizational authority, and the case manager has authority for the progression of his or her cases. Because there is an overlap in accountability, a matrix is more complex than a hierarchical organization, and the student practicing in a matrix will be accountable to both the head nurse and the case manager. As with the rest of the managed care system, the authority structure is complex. Adding another authority figure (the case manager) to the clinical domain makes an already challenging environment even more difficult, so students need to learn how to negotiate in such a complex system. They need to learn that one can be accountable to different persons for different functions, and they need to understand the importance of good interpersonal relationships to grease the wheels in such complex organizations.

Despite this organizational complexity, the case manager can be of great assistance in the education of students, in several ways. First, the case manager helps students keep their eyes on patient outcomes. For young students, having specified outcomes provides an anchor for performance, a measure by which to gauge success. Next, clinical pathways developed by a department of case management provide a student with the equivalent of a ready-made nursing care plan, with the advantage of spelling out what other professionals will do as well. Indeed, the clinical pathway gives students an opportunity to discuss their cases with other professionals. Seeking clarification of their joint roles is easier for students if they have a structure on which to base such conversations, and the clinical pathway provides it. Indeed, the presence of case management gives a defined structure to the practice environment, and this is very reassuring to students, particularly newer students.

However, faculty members may be frustrated if they are trying to reinforce a notion of professional autonomy, because autonomy may be perceived as sacrificed (or constrained) to standard operating procedures in a case management system. Still, there is a great opportunity for faculty members to teach students when it is essential to modify care and to deviate from a set plan. Hence, autonomous decision making need not be viewed as antithetical to the use of standardized clinical pathways.

The faculty may have an additional challenge if the school is implementing a particular theory of nursing, because the clinical pathway schema is itself a theory of sorts, and it is highly directive in all decision making and in all prescription of therapies. Yet the faculty member may also use this structure to point out the implications of practice for theory.

From an intellectual perspective, the faculty member will note that the system of case management (and almost any managed care strategy, for that matter) relies on "systems thinking" in which reasoning and decisions are purposely removed from the unique personalities of nurses, other health care providers, case managers, or patients. The system is highly prescriptive. In *systems thought*, each element of a plan is carefully and precisely tied to every other element in the system. See Barnum (1998, pp. 159–169) for details concerning the systems mode of thinking. The clinical pathway typifies this type of thinking, with its goals and tasks specified, usually on a day-by-day protocol. This kind of thinking may be contrasted with the problematic method of thought advocated by some faculties and some service organizations.

Problem-solving curricula (Barnum, pp.145–158) have a different orientation from the managed care system, and it may be difficult for a faculty member to teach problematic thought in a managed care environment. However, it can be taught by focusing on outcome variances as problems, if the faculty is committed to the problem-solving method. The important philosophic and practical shift inherent in the context of managed care is toward the normative patient, the normative procedure, and the highly programmed plan of care, with constant attention to monitoring and corrective activities to keep each patient "on plan." Such a plan is typically a systems model, not a problem-oriented model.

All this is based on two complementary principles. First, is the principle that the prescribed design, in the best interest of both the patient and the system, aims for early discharge from the health care institution. The assumption is that discharge means that the patient outcome goals have been achieved. The second principle is that reduced LOS is the single greatest cost-saver available in the system. The apparent agreement on the goal (early discharge of the patient) may be misleading, however, if patients go home feeling inadequate to care for themselves, or if they go to a step-down facility where employees are unprepared to give the required care.

In contrast to this disadvantage, however, one must consider a very real achievement of managed care: reduced utilization of unnecessary services. The cost saving is a valid goal in a system where costs have previously risen uncontrolled. Where cost incentives are controlled by an accurate assessment of achievement of patient outcome goals, the system works very well.

SUMMARY

Case management is one strategy by which managed care is implemented. It features outcomes assessment and LOS management. On the provider side (particularly in acute care facilities and other inpatient facilities), case management is a feedback-control system that aims to achieve the objectives of managed care: cost-effectiveness (mainly equated with reduced LOS in inpatient facilities) and control of quality of care.

Case management provides new employment opportunities for many nurses. Case managers, usually nurses, have become important players in managed care organizations (on both the provider and the payer side) because they are ideal candidates to facilitate achievement of goals by all players in the care system.

While the specific forms of case management—and the roles of all involved parties—may change from one setting to another (particularly between payer and provider organizations), it is likely that achieving patient outcomes with efficiency will retain its prominent position at the center of the managed care system.

REFERENCES

Barnum, B. S. (1998). *Nursing theory: Analysis, application, evaluation* (5th ed.). Philadelphia: Lippincott.

Barnum, B. S., & Kerfoot, K. M. (1995). *The nurse as executive* (4th ed.). Gaithersburg, MD: Aspen. (Many of the ideas in the present chapter were expressed earlier in this book, especially in chapter 13, Case management, pp. 89–97.)

Blancett, S. S., & Flarey, D. L. (1996). *Case studies in nursing case management: Health care delivery in a world of managed care.* Gaithersburg, MD: Aspen.

Cohen, E. L., & Cesta, T. G. (1993). *Nursing case management: From concept to evaluation.* St. Louis: Mosby.

Flarey, D. L., & Blancett, S. S. (1996). *Handbook of nursing case management: Health care delivery in a world of managed care.* Gaithersburg, MD: Aspen.

Mullahy, C. M. (1995). *The case manager's handbook*. Gaithersburg, MD: Aspen.

Tahan, H. A. (1993, October). The nurse case manager in acute care settings: Job description and function. *Journal of Nursing Administration, 23*(10), 53–61.

Tahan, H. A. (1996, July–August). A ten-step process to develop case management plans. *Nursing Case Management, 1*(3), 112–120.

TEST YOUR UNDERSTANDING

Multiple-Choice
Select the one *best* answer.

1. *What is the* chief *function of the case manager?*
    a. To ensure that a caseload of patients will achieve predetermined outcome goals in set time frames.
    b. To determine what care is reimbursable.
    c. To make sure that all professionals cooperate in making their plans of care.

2. *When a case management system is initiated, which kinds of patients (by diagnostic group) are typically the focus of the first clinical pathways?*
    a. Patients with the most unusual conditions.
    b. Patients who utilize the most resources.
    c. Patients who have multiple and complex diagnoses.
    d. Patients who will require extensive teaching.

3. *What is a clinical pathway?*
    a. A description of a case manager's authority in any given organization.
    b. A set of normative data, giving the institution's outcome "scorecard."
    c. A plan of patient care, including therapies, time frames, and desired outcomes.

4. *Where do case managers work?*
    a. Exclusively in provider agencies, from hospitals to skilled care facilities to long-term-care facilities.
    b. In both provider-managed and payer-managed agencies.
    c. Exclusively in payer organizations, including various insurers and employers.

5. *What is the chief role of the case manager?*
    a. To achieve predetermined outcomes with careful use of resources.
    b. To set patient care outcome goals.
    c. To process data for insurance purposes.

Discussion of Answers

1. a. This is the correct answer.
   b. Some payer case managers may have this function, but it is only a small portion of their job, and not the most important factor.
   c. The case manager is likely to deal with many professionals, but seeing that they cooperate with each other is not his or her major function.

2. a. Focusing on unusual cases would not be economically beneficial in a beginning system.
   b. This is the correct answer.
   c. These patients will require more complex clinical paths, with much variance. That complexity makes this a poor place to begin creating protocols.
   d. Because extensive teaching needs would include patients with different diagnoses, this would not be a useful place to begin creating clinical pathways.

3. a. Clinical pathways do not concern a case manager's authority.
   b. Clinical pathways are not reports of cumulative results.
   c. This is the correct answer.

4. a. This is only one setting in which case management is found.
   b. This is the correct answer.
   c. This is only one setting in which case management is found.

5. a. This is the correct answer.
   b. Usually the case manager works with care outcomes set by professionals.
   c. Some case managers may process data, but that is not their chief objective.

4

Principles Underlying Managed Care

The principles of managed care can and should inform any nursing curriculum offered today. Whether or not one prefers managed care over earlier systems, it is the dominant organizing form in most of today's health care agencies across the nation. Graduates of all nursing programs, with few exceptions, will be employed by, or interface with, institutions operating under managed care plans. The objective here is *not* to make faculty members conform unthinkingly to a managed care system, or even to make them prefer such a system. Instead, the aim is to help faculty members understand managed care and how it intimately affects the practice of all nurses operating in, or coordinating with, the system.

The premise of this book is that the teacher has an obligation to prepare students to cope with the extant health care system—good, bad, or indifferent. The faculty should explain and demonstrate how quality of care can best be achieved and maintained in the system under which the student is likely to graduate and practice.

Learning to make the best of a system in no way limits the options of reformers who want to change the system. Indeed, one might say that knowledge of an extant system is the first step in replacing it with something better. In truth, all systems change with time, and a nursing faculty should aim to instill in every student flexibility and the ability to adjust to changing care environments and changing care delivery systems.

This book, then, is neutral, recognizing managed care as the system of the moment, recognizing also that historically systems come and go, and that nursing has always had to adjust to the society and environment in which it finds itself. These chapters are designed to extract the underlying principles in managed care rather than provide the details of the system itself. It is these principles that should be considered in preparing curricula and learning experiences; it is these principles that need to be passed on to students.

Understanding the basic principles of managed care is important for nurses who will give care in today's systems as well as for those who will manage care. The early chapters provide patient care applications; subsequent chapters show how principles of managed care apply to nursing management. All this content is set in a historical context that perceives managed care as the system of the moment, taking its place in the parade of systems that have solved problems of care delivery in the past.

HISTORICAL PERSPECTIVE

Managed care is not the first system of health care delivery to be used in this country, and it will probably not be the last. On the whole, it has replaced a system that is often identified by its financial principle, that is, payment for services rendered. Managed care is also identified by its financial impetus: prospective payment in various plans designed to reward institutions that contain and control costs.

Whatever else may be said about the system of managed care, it is clearly based on a notion of health care as an economic product—more so, many would argue, than any prior orientation. Previous systems of care delivery primarily addressed health as a right (from the patient's perspective) and as a dedicated service (from the provider's perspective), with little orientation toward how the delivery system allocated and spent its resources. With uncontrolled escalation of costs, health care delivery inevitably became a major economic concern. *Economics* is "the social science that deals with the production, distribution, and consumption of goods and services" (American Heritage College Dictionary, p. 434), and from this perspective health is seen as a product to be treated in the same way as other goods and services.

As costs of health care continued to spiral upward, it was also inevitable that health would come to be perceived as a social concern that required a sharper eye to the effective and efficient allocation of resources. Today's cost containment has been achieved primarily through decreasing patients' length of stay in any institution, and through brokering various capitation plans that pay prospectively for anticipated usage of facilities and services by contracting for groups of consumers.

Managed care was implemented after the sociopolitical judgments of the larger society deemed medical care to be too costly, consuming too much of the gross domestic product. Whether or not that judgment was correct matters little at this point; the fact is that systems were put into place to cut back resources devoted to the delivery of health care. As happens with any major change in a system, the implementation of the resultant managed care system caused many disjunctures, chief among them the introduction of *economics* as one primary factor in decision making and *competition* among providers as a normal way of life. In essence, under managed care, provision of health care services became a business.

Adjustments to the new system caused each profession to go through its own change of operations, and its own trauma. Nursing was no exception—in fact, some might argue this was the profession most affected by the change. (Other professions, of course, would make the same claim.) To understand the effect of managed care on nursing, it is useful to step back and observe how nursing has adjusted to other historical changes in the health care environment. In fact, nursing has always adjusted to the environment in which it found itself. Figure 4.1 shows the pattern by which nursing has adjusted through various eras (Barnum & Kerfoot, 1995, pp. 82–88).

The pattern begins, as nursing began in this country, with *private duty:* one nurse to one patient. Originally the private duty nurse was in the patient's home. Typically, the nurse's work week involved continuous service, around the clock, for the duration of the patient's illness. Of course, the nurse probably had part of the day off each Sunday to go to church. In essence, before World War II, one could say that the *case method* prevailed. Even a nursing student did everything for the patient.

Two principles can be observed here. First, when possible, nurses prefer a *patient orientation* to a task orientation. Second, the use of nurses correlates with their *cost.* In these early days, nurses received minimal salaries. Indeed, a full-time nurse cost little more than a laundress and probably less than a good cook. In other words, nursing was cost-effective at the one-nurse-to-one-patient ratio: cheap at the price.

The Depression and changing times were responsible for a shift in the employment setting. When many people were unable to pay for nursing services in the home, nurses sought out employment in the fast-growing hospital industry. Even though hospitals, rather than homes, became the primary location of care during an illness, private duty nursing remained the pattern of care delivery; wealthier patients took their own nurses with them into hospitals. Again, the pattern of care was one nurse to one patient. The following analysis will focus on the acute care facility, although the same trends worked their way "down" the system into skilled care facilities, nursing homes, and other care delivery systems.

The pattern changed when nurses marched off to World War II with our troops, leaving a shortage of nurses on the home front. Here we see the next principle arise: a shortage of nurses usually is solved by a shift to a

Focus on patient

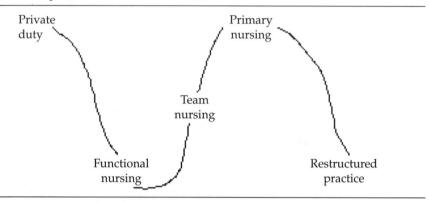

Focus on tasks

FIGURE 4.1   Nursing variables over time.

task orientation—dividing work into tasks. That is exactly what happened, and hospitals changed to meet the stressful situation. *Functional nursing* was created to get the most done with the fewest nurses. This method was modeled on the factory system of division of labor. There was a medicine nurse, a treatment nurse, a bathing nurse, and so forth. Adopting a task orientation meant that fewer nurses could take care of a greater number of patients.

One of the reasons for the change to a task orientation was the need for increased *efficiency.* A task orientation focuses on increased efficiency; in contrast, a patient orientation focuses on enhanced *effectiveness.* In this respect, the two systems have different controlling values. Effectiveness can be described as the achievement of set goals, while efficiency can be described as achievement of goals with the least use of resources. Unfortunately, efficiency sometimes gets interpreted merely as streamlining and making things move faster. Such speeding up is actually irrelevant if the goals are not achieved. For example, if we increase patients seen in a clinic by one third, yet all the patients leave confused as to what they should do now that they are leaving the clinic site, this can hardly be called efficient. Similarly, in today's cost-conscious environment it makes little sense to tout one's effectiveness in isolation from what costs and efforts went into the achievement.

When there is a change to a task orientation, another principle comes into play: *specialization.* In this early case, specialization had to do with the task assigned rather than the skill required. All RNs had the requisite skills for all the specialized tasks (e.g., passing medications, doing treatments, giving baths). Often one day's treatment nurse became the next day's medication nurse. Nevertheless, some nurses had their favorite roles, and some managed to function as specialists in those roles as often as possible.

Another practice that inevitably follows a transition to a task orientation is the use of *assistive personnel*. When task distribution is the name of the game, it is evident that different levels of skill are required for different nursing tasks. On the face of it, not all tasks require the same degree of training. Use of nurses' aides and orderlies grew during the era of functional nursing so that the work time of RNs could be husbanded for the more skilled functions.

Another principle underlying methods of care delivery is the fact that each method *solves a major problem* (or problems) presented by the previous delivery system, while itself *creating a new problem* or set of problems. For example, functional nursing solved the problem of shortage by putting efficiency before effectiveness. Later, team nursing was created to solve the problem of patients' falling through the cracks of the assembly line ideology that characterized functional nursing.

Thus, subsequent to functional nursing, *team nursing* was developed to give nurses a meaningful sense of product. In this system, a group of nurses and nurses' assistants shared the care of a small group of patients. Instead of identifying the job as a constant line of medications passed or treatments given, the nurse could recognize "Mr. Green" as her product. Patients became people again, instead of room numbers. The nurse could get to know the small number of patients on his or her "team" and could see them through their hospitalization, to a return to normal living (or to a peaceful death).

Although team nursing "cured" the problem of alienation from the patient caused by functional nursing, it brought its own set of problems. First was the fact that it did not fully escape from a task orientation to a patient orientation. The team leader still had to figure out who would do what tasks, because the team members involved had different levels of skill. Typically a team consisted of nonprofessionals and professionals, and the professionals tended to change from day to day. For example, RN Smith, as well as caring for his or her own caseload, would care for RN Black's patients on Black's day off. Tasks also varied by professional level rather than by patient, and RN Smith would still have to give medications to patients on the team assigned to nurses' aide Jones.

Furthermore, in some formulations of teams, no one had the same patients from one day to the next. Indeed, sometimes the team to which one was assigned varied from day to day, further confounding the problems which team nursing was designed to solve. Then as today, every form of assignment, no matter what its good points, could be applied ineffectively, creating new problems without solving the problems that the method was designed to cure if used effectively.

Several things happened to make team nursing more or less outdated. One was the fact that assistive personnel unionized sooner and more effectively than professional nurses. This meant that RNs suddenly became a "better buy." If an RN could "do everything," and he or she cost only slightly more than an aide, then it made sense to hire the RN.

Suddenly, we were well on the way toward the next method of care delivery: *primary nursing.* In primary care, each patient is assigned to his or her "own" RN, who is accountable for planning 24-hour care and, when on duty, for delivering that care. Each RN has a permanent caseload of patients that he or she retains until their discharge from the facility or system. Nurses loved this system, of course, because it represented a return to the patient orientation, their preferred model. The nurse was once again assigned to patients, not to tasks. (Primary nursing, an assignment system, should not be confused with primary care—the initial diagnosis and treatment of a patient.)

Primary nursing solved at least one of the problems that inevitably arose with team nursing—the difficulty of finding out, at any given time, who was doing what for whom. Indeed, the lack of communication and clear lines of authority was reflected in that era's familiar phrase, "I don't know; he's not on my team."

In the continuing cycle from patient orientation to task orientation and back again, another principle rears its head: *increasing complexity.* In one sense, primary nursing was a return to private duty, but with more complexities, more bells and whistles. Although each patient now had his or her own nurse (a recycling of the one-to-one model), few nurses had only one patient. In this era, unlike the old days, the nurse had a caseload. On the other hand, nurses did not work 24-hour, 7-day weeks. The nurse now had days off, vacations, education days, and sick time; in that they were not constantly present, primary nurses did not resemble the old private duty nurse.

In fact, primary nursing was an accountability structure more than a model for care assignments. Individual patients had their "own" nurse, who planned their care, but when the primary nurse wasn't around (which was most of the time—at least two out of three shifts each day), someone else delivered the actual care. Once again, with primary nursing the task-orientation model receded, assistive personnel were decreased, and the notion of *professional staffing* became popular, often interpreted as an essential component of primary nursing.

The primary care model held sway until the environment once again changed. If price had made primary nursing and professional staffing popular, price was what made both of them fade. At the peak of these trends, nurses broke the salary barrier in a big way. Nurses at Columbia University, for example, negotiated salaries upward to $50,000. Other institutions quickly followed. Thus RNs were no longer the best buy for the dollar.

Furthermore, the principle of scarcity once again took hold. This time, scarcity was created not by a lack of available nurses but by a reduction in the number of nurses that institutions could afford to hire, given the rising salaries of RNs and the new game of cost-driven managed care. That the new scarcity took nurses by surprise was itself surprising. The profession should have calculated that, in an inelastic industry under pressure to reduce costs, there could be no other response to increased nursing salaries than to hire fewer nurses.

Where managed care is effectively implemented, it balances the two principles of economy and quality of care. Indeed, if one takes the long view, it can be argued that these two principles do not conflict. Yet, as many nurses see it, in practice quality often has been sacrificed to economy (Baer, Fagin, & Gordon, 1996). Whatever the potential for a good balance, many nurses have found themselves in systems where economy seems to have priority, and examples of flaws in care are often publicized.

One thinks, for example, of a highly renowned hospital where patients were dismissed from one-day surgery immediately after procedures known to place the patient at risk of urinary retention. The institution tells these patients to return if a problem arises. The institution claims that this practice creates a major cost savings because only about 10 to 15% of the patients will develop the problem. To house 100% of these patients until voiding has been assured was seen as an unnecessary expense. From the institution's perspective, this makes sense. Unfortunately, this is a hospital that services patients who may have come from great distances; thus many were required to stay in local hotels, waiting to see if they belonged to the 10 to 15%, before beginning a long journey home. Did cost efficiency displace quality of care in this example (which is a typical one)? One could make an argument on both sides.

Managed care, for good or ill, has arrived, and nursing has to adapt or place its practitioners in an impossible situation. In this environment (characterized internally by decreased monies with which to hire nurses and constant demands for ever-increasing cost savings while meeting the outcome goals for more acute patients faster), it was essential that nursing reorganize its delivery system.

As always happens in a shortage (an environment of *resource scarcity*), the focus shifts from a patient orientation to a task orientation. *Restructured practice*—under its many different names, such as *differentiated practice* and *reengineered practice*—became the method of choice. If the systems were created with sophistication and good planning, the restructuring typically involved examining and recasting all professional and other service roles in an institution. At worst, the nursing department struggled to restructure nursing practice alone.

The principles of restructured practice were not unlike the principles ruling an earlier system of task-oriented nursing—functional nursing. The focus was on who should do what task, and this was decided according to level of skill. Once again, the use of unlicensed assistive personnel (UAPs) became popular. This time, however, the job definitions for UAPs were not universal but were tailored on the spot according to the needs of the individual system. New constellations of job activities created UAP positions that were quite different from the old nurses' aide jobs. The job titles (e.g., coronary care nursing technician, orthopedic technician) reflected these differences. The age of specialization had drifted down to the unlicensed level of personnel, and not all UAPs were prepared for the same functions.

Specialization, even at the technician level, was only one way in which the new task-oriented system was more complex than its forerunner, functional nursing. By now, professional nurse specialist roles, de facto, had become so dissimilar that nurses could no longer easily be substituted for each other in various areas of an institution. The obstetric nurse was not of much use in the emergency room, and the orthopedic nurse could do little in the coronary care unit.

In restructured practice, flexible use of staff sometimes was encouraged by cross-training among and between specialists, among and between adjacent units, and even among and between employees of different professions—a practice that could be seen as calling everyone's license into question.

Further, since managed care made decreasing the length of a patient's stay a fiscal mandate, complex and standardized clinical pathways and protocols of care were coming into fashion, tied to standard therapies and planned time schedules in which desired outcomes were to be achieved. Nurses, and often physicians and other professionals as well, were being forced into an uncomfortable uniformity of practice that tended to censure and penalize any practitioner who was different and who made more demands on the system's resources.

In addition to the creation, implementation, evaluation, and revision of hundreds or thousands of clinical pathways, this task-oriented system was more complex than its task-oriented predecessor in another way: a patient orientation was superimposed on top of the task-oriented system through the oversight role of the case manager. Here was a role whose incumbent looked at a caseload of patients as individuals who were making, or failing to make, progress toward programmed goals.

Indeed, we can modify the original Figure 4.1 into a two-tailed model, representing this added complexity. For the first time one sees the potential for a somewhat equal focus on patients (outcomes, goals) and on tasks.

In the old functional system, this knitting-together function was performed only by the head nurse, whose singular role offered a view of the whole operation, a perspective on the progress of all patients. In today's system, with more patients under more protocols and more deadlines, the linking function became critical. With capitation, an institution was vulnerable to

Focus on patient

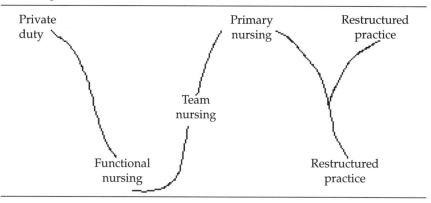

FIGURE 4.2 **Nursing variables over time.**

financial loss if a patient was slow to achieve goals, in other words, if the patient remained in the facility longer than absolutely necessary. Length of stay was critical; goals were set for achievement in the shortest feasible time.

Thus case management was invented (or, more accurately, borrowed from public health). Case management gave the nursing profession a very powerful role (in those organizations where case managers were nurses) because the role included a *gatekeeper* function, often for other professions as well as for nursing. Because the case manager interfaces with all the professionals involved in a patient's care and monitors their performance, he or she has clout beyond the nursing sphere. The case manager does for patients what the head nurse used to do—knits their care together.

As can be seen in this review of changing management systems within nursing care, change is inevitable and dictated by the external environment. In creating restructured practice and interfacing its roles with the roles of other professionals, nursing was once again responding to a set of external pressures. Numerous changes can be identified as crucial in this latest adjustment: (1) a task orientation, (2) a focus on efficiency, (3) cost-consciousness, (4) a systems design, and (5) interprofessional coordination.

EDUCATIONAL IMPLICATIONS

Clinical Students

To be contemporary, a faculty designing basic or advanced clinical curricula should set the orientation to any nursing role in a context of comprehensive health care, not an insular nursing context. While this may place a burden on the faculty, it is a fact that under the managed care structure the nurse has become a member of a care team. This is epitomized by the role of case manager, but all roles now require cooperative team performance. Nurses and other team members are playing by a set of rules determined by cost containment, limited resources, and competition.

Basic principles of managed care should be presented to clinical students, as well as the effects of these principles on nursing care delivery. Giving basic students details of numerous managed care plans may be counterproductive—the students may lose the dominant concepts among all the diversity. Clarity on just how the system works is the ideal.

Beyond managed care as content, it is important that faculty members themselves learn to look at nursing as a business. No amount of content on managed care will supplant the faculty member's own orientation to care delivery as a business. In other words, inculcation is the chief way that students learn how the system works. If the faculty member thinks from a business perspective, the student will learn to do the same.

Inculcation can be as basic as calling students' attention to their own cost-effective use of time, for example, or calling their attention to procedures and practices that have been changed to save costs. If the faculty member takes a negative view of nursing as a business, the student is likely to pick up this attitude, no matter what aspects of managed care are officially included as course content.

Faculty members, then, must work through their own feelings about the fact that nursing and health care are now conducted as businesses. In truth, whether a given system has successfully blended cost and quality objectives, the faculty member in the clinical domain has an excellent opportunity to demonstrate instances when both goals can be served simultaneously. To fail to prepare students for this reality does them a disservice.

The curriculum also can present a business orientation toward health care in general, that is, as one value among many over which a society must distribute its scarce resources. This viewpoint is quite different from the traditional philosophy underlying most nursing curricula, that is, that health and health care are values beyond price. Today they have a price, and students unprepared to recognize that fact will be at a distinct disadvantage when they try to understand what is happening in an institution. Nor will naive students be able to uphold the position of nursing in the internal organizational competition for resources.

Student also should be taught to see other professionals in both cooperative and competitive modalities. The truth is that resources given to nursing are resources removed from some other sector of a melded body of corporate interests. The blending of interorganizational competition for resources with cooperative mutual patient care practice calls for a sensitive balance.

Because new delivery systems force the nurse to oversee diverse personnel, three more essentials enter the basic education of nurses. First, they must learn two aspects of *delegation*. The first concerns what can be delegated to whom. A nursing curriculum should include criteria by which to distribute tasks downward safely. For example, which tasks are routine and which are likely to require that judgments be made while implementing them? Which tasks have the potential for changing the patient's status negatively if ill-performed? Which tasks require modifications in each case? After one considers the logic of what can be delegated, one must still balance decisions against the legal implications of delegation. State licensure laws must be included in any determination of delegation.

In addition to discussing the *content* of delegation, clinical students need to become familiar with the *process* of delegation. Clinical practice is essential to internalize the principles of delegation. Young students, for example, may need to develop confidence before they can comfortably delegate assignments to nurses' aids who know the system better than the students and who possibly recognize the students' vulnerabilities as well.

It is also essential for the clinical student to learn about *supervision* and *evaluation* of a group of care delivery employees. Clinical experience, even for generic students, should include the management and evaluation of subordinate unlicensed and licensed employees as well as supervision of peers, superordinates, and other professionals. Supervisory skills include but are not limited to these basics: making clear assignments, telling an employee what is expected, periodically observing and reviewing the employee's progress, and giving feedback and correction.

Curricula also should give principles by which to evaluate the employee's performance. Students should be taught how to locate and use the organizational documents that describe the requisite skills of a staff, from UAPs to other professionals (e.g., social workers). Because students may be insecure in evaluating personnel who have different or more advanced capacities than their own, outcomes assessment should be taught—it is a valuable tool in this effort.

These few comments cannot convey all that a student needs to know about delegation, supervision, and evaluation, each element of which could constitute a short course on its own. However, the faculty member should get a sense of how important these process skills are for students if they are to function in today's managed care systems.

In recent years, most vestiges of management were removed from clinical curricula. Indeed, in the era of primary nursing care, these managerial skills were less important. In an era of managed care, however, managerial process skills again become critical.

The student's perspective on the patient also will be modified, changing past images. Whenever possible, patients should be presented as consumers as well as recipients of health care. Competition for patient dollars should be linked to services delivered, as well as patients' perceptions and choices. Although clinical students need not know all there is to know about managed care, they do need an orientation to the system and the expectations it implies for the patient and the nurse.

Nursing Administration Students

Although all curricula for nursing administration students today are likely to give considerable detail concerning managed care in many of its formulations, it is essential that the principles underlying the system be emphasized. Processes essential to operating and decision making within such a cost-driven system must be included as preparation for administrative roles. Fiscal implications of managed care should include those items expected of every manager in today's system, from variance analysis, budgeting, cost-benefit analysis, and cost-effectiveness analysis to the creation of business plans. The ability to put together a business plan for a proposed administrative change is an essential competitive tool today. It is an excellent way for students to appreciate the interplay of quality care and cost factors.

Nursing administration students should be given theories of contextual management, along with criteria by which to assess the current environment. Environmental assessment is a required process, inherent in strategic planning (which will be discussed in later chapters). In short, the nursing administration student must be grounded not only in the theories of managed care but in the concrete application of its strategies and tactics.

SUMMARY

Everyone recognizes that the principles of cost savings and quality of care underlie the managed care system; yet there are less-evident principles that also hold for the system. The principles included a predominant *task orientation* over a patient orientation, and that leads to a matching of worker skill level to tasks performed. This evolves into the principle dominant in a factory model, that is, *division of labor* by tasks. A principle related to cost saving is one of *sparse use of expensive resources,* and that includes costly personnel. Division of labor leads to growth of role *specialization* as well.

Return of these principles means that students must once again receive education in the management of other personnel. A singular nursing role model no longer is adequate. Skills such as supervision, delegation, and personnel evaluation become an essential part of the basic nursing role. Management skills are an inherent part of the nurse's role under managed care.

REFERENCES

The American heritage college dictionary. (1993). Boston: Houghton Mifflin.

Baer, E. D., Fagin, C. M., & Gordon, S. (Eds.). (1996). *Abandonment of the patient: The impact of profit-driven health care on the public.* New York: Springer.

Barnum, B. S., & Kerfoot, K. M. (1995). *The nurse as executive* (4th ed.). Gaithersburg, MD: Aspen. (Much of the material in the present chapter was adapted from chap. 12, pp. 82–88.)

TEST YOUR UNDERSTANDING

Multiple-Choice

Select the one *best* answer.

1. *Which new element dominates decisions about care delivery today?*
    a. Quality of care.
    b. Consumers' financial status.
    c. Cost containment.
    d. Patients' insurance coverage.

2. *Which principle accounts for nursing's recent change to restructured practice?*
    a. Surplus of nurses.
    b. Effectiveness.
    c. Efficiency.
    d. Task orientation.

3. *What is the best way to describe the value of the managed care system?*
    a. Better than all prior systems of health care management.
    b. Designed to deliver in a time of demand for economy.
    c. Allows each profession to practice at its peak.
    d. Gives patients more equitable access.

4. *What is the best system of nursing care delivery?*
    a. Primary nursing with professional staffing.
    b. Team nursing modifications.
    c. No system is ever better than any other.
    d. Whatever system fits its health care environment.

5. *What is the chief characteristic of the role of nursing case manager?*
    a. Patient orientation.
    b. Focus on task completion.
    c. Interprofessional cooperation.
    d. New hierarchical management.

Discussion of Answers

1. a. Quality of care is of major importance for every health care professional; it is our reason for being. However, quality of care is not the new element that structures most of today's health care system.
    b. Consumers' status is being taken into account these days in many ways, including differentiated care according to various levels of

payment. However, this is not the primary driving force of today's system.

   c. This is the correct answer.

   d. Patients' insurance coverage may determine whether or not they are admitted to an agency (except in emergencies, life-threatening situations). However, this is not the dominant element in decisions about care delivery today.

2. a. A surplus of nurses in an organization would be likely to lead to a patient-oriented system, not a restructured one.

   b. Effectiveness places qualitative factors first, and restructured practice requires quantitative factors.

   c. This is the correct answer.

   d. Nurses seldom prefer a task orientation. They adopt such an orientation only when there is no other fit.

3. a. Managed care cannot be called a "better" system unless one establishes criteria determining what constitutes "best."

   b. This is the correct answer.

   c. "Peak" implies that quality is more dominant than cost containment. This probably does not represent most of managed care today.

   d. Managed care may make for inequitable access, with discrimination shown against patients who have orphan diseases or lack insurance coverage.

4. a. Primary care may be a nurse's preference, but the system has its own limitations. For example, if one's primary nurse is inadequate there may be few others around to pick up the deficit.

   b. Modified team is a popular choice, but it too has its own limitations. For example, team leaders may not be prepared for the staff management expectations of their roles.

   c. Systems are not absolutes; they must be considered in context.

   d. This is the correct answer.

5. a. This is the correct answer.

   b. While the case manager appears in a task-oriented system, this role is not based on task completion.

   c. Interprofessional cooperation will make the case manager's role easier, but the role was not invented to improve interpersonal relations or to enhance interprofessional actions.

   d. The case manager may or may not have hierarchical managerial authority, and the roles may be structured differently in different institutions. This factor does not characterize the role.

5

The Philosophy of Total Patient Care

To fully understand the effects of managed care on nursing and on the teaching of nursing, one must first examine the beliefs that have been held by the nursing profession for long periods and with strong emotions. The most important of those beliefs is a commitment to the philosophy of *total patient care* and all that it implies. If nursing faculty members continue to hold this belief without examining it, they will be unable to deal with the changing health care system except pejoratively.

Nursing has a long history of teaching its students to provide total patient care, that is, comprehensive patient care in which the student conceptualizes, then attempts to meet, all of the patients' actual real and potential needs for health care. Until recently, every nursing student learned this ideal. Many faculty members will remember that they themselves were taught to give total patient care. Often, they pass this ideal along to their own students without considering whether or not it is appropriate.

We call total (or comprehensive) patient care idealistic because it is based on goals set in the abstract. The nurse is responsible for providing everything deemed good for the patient. For that reason, this philosophy uses a *goal-driven model* (Barnum & Kerfoot, 1995, pp. 10–14). Successful nursing care implies identifying all the potential needs of the patient, setting relevant goals for each identified need, and achieving all the goals. It would be equally accurate to call this model *needs-driven*.

Goal-driven care is basically a philosophy rather than an assignment method. It underlies an unspoken nursing value—that the "good" nurse provides for all the patient's needs. Often a faculty member is uncomfortable with the notion of providing anything less than goal-driven care because his or her professional identity has become closely associated with the delivery of excellent care, and "excellent care" has become a way of saying, "Do everything; meet every health need."

If the faculty member recognizes that ideal care is a value, it will be easier to understand the teaching implications of that position, as well as to appreciate the merits of alternative viewpoints. In the ideal care model, the value of nursing is associated with the comprehensiveness of the care. We will suggest that, alternatively, excellent nursing can be associated with giving the best possible care in the circumstances—a *contextual model* of care rather than a *content model.*

First, however, it is essential to understand the mechanism of the older, goal-driven model.

GOAL-DRIVEN NURSING

In goal-driven care, no matter what assignment method is used, one starts with the patient. The assumption is that the nurse can and will assess all the patient's needs, and that the nurse can and will set goals to meet all those needs. This holds true for every patient assigned to a nurse. In this model at its simplest, the nurse assesses the patient, identifies his or her needs, projects interventions designed to meet all those needs, implements the interventions, and evaluates the outcomes. Under this goal-driven system, the faculty member not only evaluates the quality of the student's interventions and the patient outcomes but also evaluates whether or not the student has identified all the patient's needs.

A subtle problem arises in this model if the patient or his needs differ from the nurse's perceptions or if the patient and nurse differ on what health care goals are to be achieved. Essentially, nursing has accepted the professional model: that is, the nurse is assumed to know best. Lip service is sometimes given to planning with the patient rather than for the patient, but few models actually yield control to the patient. For the rest of this discussion, we will assume the typical model in which the nurse diagnoses, sets goals, and implements the care.

Conflict of the Goal-Driven Model with Reality

In many cases the ideal level of care is not possible (or supported) in today's delivery environment; yet the notion dies hard. One version of total patient care that prevails today is nursing care determined by applying the nursing process and using *nursing diagnoses.* In this common formulation, the nurse assesses the total patient, coming up with a comprehensive list of all pertinent nursing diagnoses. These diagnoses cumulatively dictate the substance of the nursing care. Treatment plans are expected to be set for every diagnosis.

Unless this model of nursing process–nursing diagnosis is modified by a notion of prioritizing in which care is limited to high-priority items, it may be seen as today's version of total patient care. We describe this model and all total-patient-care models as *goal-driven* because they originate in perceived needs of the patient translated without mediation into desired goals and therapeutic interventions. The key defining principle of the goal-driven model is that the work flow originates in the patient, or more accurately, in the nurse's assessment of the patient. There is no notion of compromise or limitation in goal-driven models, no sense that the patient is paying only for a given amount of care, and certainly no inference that the institution has the ability to deliver only part of the package.

Yet the truth is that few institutions have the available resources, especially nursing hours, to provide all the care that might be envisioned for every patient in the system. This is the problem that arises under goal-driven models: they are effective only in ideal conditions, that is, where there are enough resources (equipment, supplies, nursing hours) to do everything. Ironically, the smarter and more thorough nurses are, the more goals they may envision; and if they envision too many, they are bound to lack the time to meet them all. This creates a situation where greater effort is rewarded with greater frustration.

Goal-driven models assume that the resources needed to deliver the comprehensive package of patient care will be forthcoming. Whether nurses have ever actually practiced under ideal circumstances is not the point. Indeed, generations of faculties have provided the ideology of ideal care as the prototype for tomorrow, as the sort of care that is always just around the corner, or worse: as the sort of care the student is challenged to make possible.

Limitations of Goal-Driven Models

Models advocating delivery of comprehensive care are vulnerable to failure when control over the nurse's environment and its resources (including time) is only partial. Moreover, nurses who have learned to equate their self-worth with the inclusiveness of their work for each patient find that they must change that idea or judge themselves to be failures. Required resources are important in calculating nursing care, and most of the resources are not supplies and equipment; they are nursing hours and, secondarily, care systems.

Nurses educated and working under a goal-driven ideology are assumed to "do everything" for a patient, and that is the sticking point.

They are vulnerable to feelings of failure unless they work in a resource-rich environment.

Several problems arise under a goal-driven ideology of care. The first has to do with not completing physician-ordered tasks. Where physicians' orders are seen as nondiscretionary, and there is not enough time to complete all the orders, nurses resort to various strategies. One strategy is to sacrifice all independent nursing measures to better serve the physician's orders. Another is the old challenge: that nurses remain "on duty" until their work is completed. Where nurses get overtime, that practice does not last long in today's environment; but students, whose time is sometimes seen as elastic, are often held to it. For the most part, nurses have now become comfortable with telling physicians when there simply are not enough hours to complete ordered therapeutics.

Administrators may assume that the clever nurse will find the resources to deliver all the work. Indeed, many nursing texts advise the nurse to "practice smarter, not faster." This is not to negate the creativity of nurses in finding extra resources and streamlining procedures, but there are very real limitations to the ways in which creativity can substitute for a lack of essential hours.

In a system of managed care, with its tight control and limitation of resources, it is not surprising that the goal-driven model may generate more goals (patient outcomes) than are envisioned in the typical clinical pathway. Goal-driven models, by their nature, generate work; managed care, by design, limits work. The logical approach is for everyone to recognize when goal-driven care is not possible and other models should be used. Chapter 6 will discuss a reasonable alternative.

EDUCATIONAL IMPLICATIONS

Because so many nurses, including faculty members, accept the goal-driven model of nursing without thinking, it is important that they learn to recognize this attitude when they see it. This can be done by making the model overt instead of covert. Simply put, faculties and students will profit from a discussion of how goals relate to resources. Students in any program can benefit from understanding their heritage—the goal-driven model. They will benefit from having the assumptions of the model explained, no matter what their curriculum.

Furthermore, beginning students probably ought to be introduced to the concept of ideal care early in their clinical practice. In a first term, they might be expected to give ideal care to one or two patients, but they should be told that their initial practice is being simplified, that because of their inexperience they are being given an artificial practice world. Just as beginners are given "simpler" patients, it makes sense to give them less time pressure, and a goal-driven model achieves this. A limited number of patients (which the instructor calculates will not create time pressures) will allow the student to be held to account for a semblance of ideal care (modified only by the student's inexperience).

Ideal care may be used for one school term at most, and never should the student be made to feel that this practice is or should be "normal." Students should understand that this is attenuated practice, for the sake of learning. Students should be made aware from the start that the world of nursing, like most other worlds of work, is seldom ideal. A student who expects the world to correspond with the ideal will inevitably be disappointed. If students are able to work only under ideal circumstances, they have been sadly unprepared for reality.

SUMMARY

Total patient care (or comprehensive patient care) is the philosophy of care that has long dominated in nursing and nursing education. Under this model, it is assumed that the nurse will meet every identifiable health need evinced by the patient. This practice can be labeled a needs-driven or a goal-driven model, because it starts with the patient, not with a consideration of external circumstances. This model may be highly unrealistic in an era of restricted resources. When nurses judge their worth by their ability to implement the total patient care model, they may be dooming themselves to negative judgments.

Because this philosophy has been accepted for so long, the goal-driven model may be applied in circumstances where the nurse is unaware that he or she is applying it. Then the nurse may become a victim of a system in which success may be impossible. Hence, the nurse should be aware of the philosophy underlying care delivery.

REFERENCES

Barnum, B. S., & Kerfoot, K. M. (1995). *The nurse as executive* (4th ed.). Gaithersburg, MD: Aspen. (Much of the material in the present chapter was adapted from chap. 2, pp. 82–88.)

TEST YOUR UNDERSTANDING

Multiple-Choice

Select the one *best* answer.

1. *How do the nursing process and nursing diagnoses relate to goal-driven models of care? Combined, they are:*
   a. A systems model, not goal-driven.
   b. A goal-driven system in themselves.
   c. Based on an entirely different philosophy.

2. *The chief advantage of goal-driven care, where it can be applied, is that:*
   a. Patients have all their needs addressed.
   b. It is less costly than other methods.
   c. It is the only method that focuses on patient outcomes.

3. *The chief limitation of goal-driven models is that:*
   a. They require a very smart nurse.
   b. They may set unattainable objectives.
   c. They discourage quality practice.

4. *For beginning nursing students, a goal-driven model represents:*
   a. A good place to start.
   b. A model to be discouraged.
   c. Class content, but never a practice orientation.

Discussion of Answers

1. a. Whether or not they are used in a systems model, it is still a goal-driven model.
   b. This is the correct answer.
   c. The philosophies are identical.

2. a. This is the correct answer.
   b. Goal-driven care tends to be more expensive because it is more expansive and uses more resources.
   c. This system is not the only one to focus on patient outcomes, as the heavy use of clinical pathways in contrasting managed care systems illustrates.

3. a. A nurse has more time and less need to prioritize or make other hard choices in goal-driven systems so any nurse can use such a model.
   b. This is the correct answer.
   c. This system fosters quality practice.

4. a. This is the correct answer.
   b. There is nothing wrong with starting with the ideal, as long as one doesn't assume that it represents reality.
   c. Class content should deal with the realities too; it should not be different from the practice situation.

6

Resource-Driven Models

Today, goal-driven care has been replaced with resource-driven care (Barnum & Kerfoot, 1995, pp. 10–14). The latter, unlike the former, is structurally compatible with managed care. In the resource-driven philosophy of nursing, one starts not with the patient but instead with the surroundings. In examining the surroundings—the environment—nurses take into account its given resources. Then they determine what goals they can reasonably take on (given their time and their assignment) for a patient or a group of patients. Required resources are important in calculating nursing care, and these resources include supplies, equipment and, primarily, nursing hours. The resources drive the goals, not the other way around.

Like managed care, the resource-driven model is context-oriented, and the context is usually one of economy, if not scarcity. Any nurse who has served in a combat zone will recognize the scarcity model: priority triage. Disaster nursing makes similar assumptions, the chief of which is to do the most critical things first when it is not possible to do everything. There have always been resource-driven models in nursing, even if emergency room nursing and disaster nursing no longer appear in many nursing curricula.

In any form of resource-driven care, environmental resources have a major impact on what one does. Decisions, sometimes hard ones, are required in selecting the best goals possible in order to get the most mileage out of resources. If resources happen to be plentiful, then one can take on more goals.

A resource-driven model can be applied to the care of a single patient, but more commonly a nurse applies it to the total package of work derived from a patient assignment, whatever that may be (e.g., assigned acute patients, clinic visits, home visits). In the resource-driven model, one considers and weighs all the potential goals for a patient cohort, prioritizes them, and decides on a feasible number of goals for enactment from the top of the list.

A resource-driven model may be applied in any setting, from an acute care hospital to a community facility to the nurse's own entrepreneurial business. A resource-driven model is setting-neutral. In each setting, one considers the resources, whether they be the hours available for a given patient load in an acute care hospital, or the number of minutes for the average clinic visit in a community setting, or the number of home care patients to be seen in a week. The quantity calculations require one to estimate and distribute the workload (available nursing time) where it will do the most good. The same is true for usage patterns of limited supplies.

A resource-driven model is more complex than a goal-driven model because it demands that one make more choices. An accurate fit must be achieved between available resources and the work to be done, that is, the goals to be taken on. If goal-driven care had its origin in factors related to quality, then resource-driven care demands a mesh of factors related to quality and quantity—not just effectiveness but efficiency as well. The chief quantity factor, because it is usually the main cost in the health care system, is the nurse's time. The first question becomes how much and what sort of care can be given with a limited number of man-hours.

Many faculty members will recall giving student assignments that entailed hours of research to complete a single nursing care plan. The students could take as much time as required. They poured everything into the care plan, being careful not to skip a single patient need or goal, because the faculty member would find that one omission. As a learning experience, an assignment like this teaches the student to be thorough, but the student must come to understand that the clinical setting is not the arena for such slow deliberation and research. A nursing faculty must acquaint students with the characteristics of the clinical arena, such as the following: (1) Many things happen at once, and the important things are not differentiated from the inconsequential. (2) Time pressure is imposed on everyone from multiple sources. (3) Demands will always be in excess of the time needed to meet them. (4) At its best, the arena is a high-stress environment. (5) Slow and leisurely deliberation must be done before or after immersion in this environment.

Today's nurse must make more complex professional decisions, determining what things to do and what things not to do for which patients. Priorities are critical: Often the nurse must make hard choices between what is essential and what is merely beneficial.

In the resource-driven model, the nurse determines potential patient goals—let us say, all the goals that might be tackled for an assignment of eight patients. There is nothing wrong with determining those goals by assessment of patients, but the depth of the assessment may itself be dictated by an initial assessment of available time.

All the goals of the patient group together will be prioritized and translated into nursing tasks (methods) required to achieve them. Then comes the quantitative part. The nurse estimates the time involved to complete these tasks and weighs it against his or her available hours. A nurse who is working with an assistant of any kind may compare it against their joint time.

If the initial task list far outweighs the available time, the nurse will start to eliminate the least essential goals and their associated tasks. Or the nurse may determine that other methods of meeting the goals would be less costly in terms of hours. A nurse working in a community care center, for example, may be able to stretch the available time by teaching groups rather than individuals, if the clients have similar learning needs. In all cases, what can be done is determined on the basis of available resources. Of course, resources can be expanded if the nurse is clever. Is there a volunteers' association, for example, that might be asked to perform nontechnical tasks? What help can be anticipated from patients' families? Could a nurse's business profit by training some home care aides to do work previously done by the nurse-owner? In all cases, reality rules, changing the determined tasks from a wish list to a feasible work assignment based on environmental constraints.

Three practical principles of resource-driven care are: (1) Work tasks are achieved over time. (2) Resources are usually perceived as set, not infinitely expandable. (3) Revised systems or streamlined methods may extend available resources.

COMPARISON OF NURSING CARE MODELS

Goal-driven and resource-driven models may be compared on many dimensions. First, their *underlying assumptions* are different. The goal-driven model assumes that all worthy goals should be tackled and that, with the proper initiative, the nurse will find the necessary resources to achieve the goals.

In contrast, the resource-driven model takes the system's resources as more or less given, expecting work to conform to the available nursing time, equipment, and supplies. Certainly creativity and cleverness may help a nurse make the best of a situation when resources are limited, but on the whole, nurses work within the available assets rather than believing that the system will provide additional ones if necessary.

Nurses often say that members of the medical profession have a god complex. If that is true, then nursing has its own complex: an angel complex. We tend to act as if any number of nurses, no matter how few, can complete a work assignment of any magnitude. Yet even on roller skates, two nurses couldn't adequately take care of a unit of 30 acute patients or double the number of clinic patients seen without loss of quality of care.

By being flexible in the methods selected to achieve goals, nurses may stretch resources in many cases. This is when they must make tough choices. Suppose one method of doing a task is comprehensive but lengthy. Is there a shorter method that is almost as good? Easily accessible hot moist packs might not be as good as whirlpool baths, but they beat no therapy at all. A computerized patient learning package may be less personal, but is it really less effective than one-on-one teaching? How much less effective? Assessments and questions like these inevitably enter into choice of methods.

The *processes* by which the two models work are significantly different also. The goal-driven model begins by setting goals derived from assessment and diagnosis of the patient. The nurse then determines the methods that will achieve the goals and implements the plan. Finally, the nurse evaluates to what extent the goals have been achieved.

In contrast, the process of resource-driven care begins with an assessment of the resources at hand. Only then is the nurse in a position to determine what goals (from a plethora of potential ones) can be achieved, given the assets. In resource-driven care, the number of goals that can be tackled may affect the assignment system. Where there are few nurses, for example, a charge nurse might select a less favored method if it is known to be a time-saver. For example, a functional care assignment method might be substituted for a primary care design in a staffing crisis. Or, in a shared partnership clinic, a nurse may need to adjust his or her patient visits to the same length as that of the physician peer to establish parity, even if this means modifying visit goals.

Evaluation also differs in the two models. In a goal-driven model, nurses simply check to see if they have achieved the predetermined patient-related goals. In the resource-driven model, there are many more aspects to be evaluated. The nurse must ask if resources were accurately defined, whether an appropriate number of goals were tackled, whether the goals were achieved, and whether the best methods were chosen.

Similarly, there are *limitations* to both methods. If the necessary resources cannot be found, the goal-driven system breaks down. If not all worthy goals can be achieved, nurses perceive themselves as a failure. Worse, if nurses attempt to do "everything" when that is impossible, critical aspects of care may be skipped haphazardly.

A limitation of the resource-driven model is that some achievable objectives may not be attempted. A miscalculation may lead a nurse to undertake less care delivery than was possible. Learning to estimate resources (especially time) is not easy. This is the point where issues of quantity and quality meet.

Another danger in the resource-driven model occurs when there simply are not enough resources for basic safe care. Because of this risk, a nurse using a resource-driven model needs a safety net, that is, clear criteria for recognizing when levels of care are unsafe. Without such indices, dangerous deficiencies may be tolerated.

Each system, goal-driven and resource-driven, has some *advantages* over the other. A goal-driven model gives the nurse the satisfaction of practicing exemplary care. Because the nursing process and its evaluation are relatively simple, this is a good model for an inexperienced nurse or a beginning student.

In the resource-driven model, however, nurses have the advantage of recognizing when they give good care even in a bad situation. Imagine an emergency when three nurses are in a rehabilitation center that should be staffed for six. If their planning and care delivery are based on a resource-based model, they can go home saying, "We couldn't do everything, but we made the best choices possible." Or imagine a clinic run by a nurse where reimbursement policies limit the time of patients' visits. While a full assessment of the patient's health knowledge may not fit into an initial visit, important assessment questions can be systematically scheduled as components of each subsequent visit. When care assignments are reality-based, it makes for a less frenetic environment where fewer mistakes may be made.

Further, the resource-driven model is adaptable. Although it is usually applied in a resource-scarce environment, it may be applied in a resource-rich environment as well. In the case of a resource-rich environment, the nurse simply takes on more goals. This is true for every setting, from acute care to home care.

THE REALITY FACTOR

Advocates of the resource-driven model would assert that excellence in nursing practice has never really been separate from its environmental resources, and expert nursing can take place in the most difficult of circumstances. Nightingale did not find the best of all possible worlds in Scutari. Excellence consists of optimizing the possible; simply put, it is what one does with what one has. A model that demands that nurses find the necessary resources to deliver perfect care without consideration of cost may be unrealistic in our era of managed care.

On the other hand, working with a resource-driven model does not preclude simultaneously seeking to enhance one's resources. As one learns to make intelligent decisions in the resource-driven model, one gains experience in weighing and balancing issues of quality and quantity. In essence, a resource-driven model teaches the nurse to estimate with accuracy what sort of nursing may be achieved with a given number of resources. Weighing costs and benefits becomes second nature.

Because it works on the same principles as managed care (balancing quality and quantity), resource-driven nursing care is compatible with general managed care. Both systems work on the basis of cost-benefit and cost-effectiveness models. Cost-benefit models provide a balance scale with which to compare the costs and benefits of a given process or administrative plan. Cost-effectiveness models, by contrast, enable one to see what sort of goals can be achieved at what level of costs. Both models typify the thinking in resource-driven care and managed care.

EDUCATIONAL IMPLICATIONS

A nursing faculty can best prepare students for today's practice by teaching them to function in an environment where there are more pressures for the students' time and attention than can be met. Hence, a student in the second term and subsequent terms of clinical experience should be introduced to the notion of quantity care as well as quality care. This can be done by teaching the resource-driven model as class content, while increasing the number of patients assigned to the student, whether they be acute care or clinic clients. The same effect can be produced by assigning the same number of patients, but selecting those with a larger number of time-consuming needs.

Clinical conferences should include discussion of time and resource management as well as clinical content, and the students should be taught to assess their effectiveness and growth in dealing with a continuously demanding environment. Discussion of pressures and choices will be important. Acquainting students with cost-benefit and cost-effectiveness models provides an intellectual underpinning for such discussions.

Clinical faculty members, obviously, have a more difficult task today than in the past. They must assess many factors in order to judge a student's performance. These factors include the student's ability to prioritize and to assess timing, the student's choice of methods, and the more traditional aspects: patient assessment, quality of intervention skills, and actual patient outcomes.

Faculty members will also have to help students remain secure if they are practicing under the resource-driven model while interfacing with a nursing staff imbued with the goal-driven model. This is true even when the staff is itself unsuccessful in implementing a goal-driven model but is still ideologically committed to it. Most important, if the faculty members themselves are uncomfortable with the resource-driven model, then students will sense this attitude and will have a difficult time applying the model. Managed care applies a business perspective to the delivery of care, and the faculty will have to imbue the student with this ideology. Often, faculty members—still in rebellion and yearning for the past—will present a managed care environment to the student in a negative way, creating in students a yearning for an idyllic past that probably never existed except in a faculty member's retrospectively revised memories.

SUMMARY

Managed care is the managerial equivalent of a resource-driven model of patient care. Both systems consider two factors: resources (costs and time) and goals to be achieved. Both are context-driven rather than focused exclusively on goals. Nor should these systems be eschewed on the basis of the "reality factor." We do not work or live in a world of infinite resources.

REFERENCES

Barnum, B. S., & Kerfoot, K. M. (1995). *The nurse as executive* (4th ed.). Gaithersburg, MD: Aspen. (Much of the material in the present chapter was adapted from chap. 2, pp. 10–14.)

TEST YOUR UNDERSTANDING

Multiple-Choice

Select the one *best* answer.

1. *Why are many nurses uncomfortable with the idea of resource-driven care?*
   a. It is a more complex model.
   b. It means admitting that not everything may be doable.
   c. Most nurses believe that any good system starts with the patient's needs.

2. *In a perfect environment (all the staff and resources one could want), which model of delivery would provide the best care?*
   a. Goal-driven care.
   b. Resource-driven care.
   c. No difference.

3. *What is the* chief *danger in resource-driven care?*
   a. Alone, it doesn't define when a dangerous lack of resources exists.
   b. It encourages nurses to think about tasks to be done rather than about patient's needs.
   c. It conflicts with nursing's philosophy of providing everything a patient may need.

4. *What is the chief reason for using resource-driven care?*
   a. It allows nurses to feel satisfied with their work in a bad situation.
   b. It saves costs for the institution.
   c. Critical tasks get done when hard choices must be made.

Discussion of Answers

1. a. It is true that this is a more complex model, but that is seldom the factor that makes nurses uncomfortable.
   b. This is the correct answer.
   c. There is nothing wrong with starting with the patient's needs, but the notion that the system starts elsewhere probably isn't the factor that elicits the most emotional response.

2. a. Goal-driven would not be better than resource-driven, since both would do "everything" in a resource rich environment.
   b. Resource-driven would not be better than goal-driven, since both would do "everything" in a resource rich environment.
   c. This is the correct answer.

3. a. This is the correct answer.
   b. This system may focus the nurse more on tasks, but that is not its chief danger.
   c. Whether or not the nurse likes the resource-driven model, the attitude itself does not present a danger.

4. a. It is important for nurses to feel satisfied with their performance, but that is not the most critical reason for using the system.
   b. Resource-driven care may be compatible with cost savings, but this is not its chief virtue.
   c. This is the correct answer.

7

Models in Nursing Management

M uch of what is presented in this chapter will have direct application in teaching students of nursing administration. However, teachers of clinical students should also appreciate facets of nursing administration in an era when clinical care and management are so intricately woven together. This chapter examines two basic goal-driven and resource-driven models of nursing administration: management by objectives and strategic management (Barnum & Kerfoot, 1995, pp. 12–20; Barnum, 1998, pp. 219–229). Each has its counterpart, respectively, in the goal-driven or resource-driven care delivery system, as well as its conflict or compatibility with the more general structure of managed care systems. Although it is not essential that the care model and the management model match in an organization, consistency among formats simplifies operations.

In an era of shrinking resources and rapidly shifting opportunities, management models are changing to fit the new reality. Management by objectives (MBO) is being replaced by strategic management as the *predominant* model. This is not to say that MBO is to be discarded. The answer in today's environment is probably a balance of strategic planning and MBO. Management by objectives can be used when the environment is predictable; strategic planning may be used when there is less predictability. We'll look at both basic models, starting with MBO.

MANAGEMENT BY OBJECTIVES

The preferred managerial approach in the era when goal-driven nursing prevailed was the traditional *management by objectives*, with yearly to five-year objectives, accompanied by careful and detailed plans for their achievement. Management by objectives is a goal-driven model of care in which one begins by setting goals—ideal ones, determined in the abstract. The managerial question was, "What do we want to achieve?" not, "What are we able to do?" True, the goals are managerial rather than patient-related, but the planning process is identical.

After setting objectives, the nurse manager (who may be anyone from a nursing vice president to a head nurse) draws up logical plans for achieving the goals, identifying what resources must be found to make the achievement possible. The plans are subjected to a formalized schedule with achievement target dates assigned at each step. The plans are implemented, then evaluated periodically and terminally.

The MBO model assumes a stable world where things do not change very much or very fast—a world where the variables are known, where one can predict the result of implementing action Q instead of action R. The world of MBO is not designed to handle unexpected curves once a plan is set into motion. Thus MBO worked best in earlier eras, where the manager could predict the future for the period of time under review.

Nursing Organizations and MBO

Management by objectives is still applied in most nursing agencies, although it has lost its place as the preferred format. Objectives are established at the top level of the nursing agency, then filtered down to lower departments and units where they are adapted and added to unit-specific objectives. If the nursing agency is part of a larger corporation, its mission (a broad statement of the division's vision and direction) is consonant with the corporation's mission.

Permanent and temporary objectives flow from mission statements. *Permanent objectives* represent those ongoing goals that must be achieved continuously, over and over again. A typical list of permanent nursing objectives might contain statements like the following:

1. Advance the practice of clinical nursing within the division.
2. Implement new research findings in clinical nursing.
3. Provide adequate resources for implementation of nursing care to meet standards of patient care.
4. Foster an environment that encourages staff members' research, creativity, inquiry, and personal growth.
5. Retain a staff that is up to date in its knowledge, application, and conceptualization of nursing practice.
6. Maintain productive relationships with other divisions and departments of the institution.
7. Contribute productively to interdisciplinary research and education.

Temporary objectives are a bridge between MBO and strategic management; they use the principle of focus and selected items for special attention in a given time period. Temporary objectives are selected to bolster known weak spots, enhance strengths, or respond to critical changes in the organization's environment. Some examples follow:

1. Improve "patient quality management" scores by 10 percent.
2. Implement a system of making the head nurse accountable for unit costs.
3. Reorganize the nursing office for achieving greater managerial efficiency with less personnel.

Temporary objectives are one-time events, supplanted by others once they have been achieved. Permanent objectives tend to be set in the traditional MBO format, while temporary objectives often arise from strategic planning. This is not to say that one-time-only objectives might not also arise under the MBO model.

SELECTING OBJECTIVES

In the MBO model, some groups have difficulty rejecting any worthy objectives. This leads to two problems: selecting more objectives than any program can reasonably attain, and selecting objectives that are mutually incompatible. If a program tries to do everything it sees as worthy, diffusion of effort and lack of direction result. Management by objectives, like goal-driven nursing, may take on too many goals.

Although MBO has faded as the preferred or exclusive management tool, the notion is highly compatible with today's focus on outcomes management. While the vocabulary may change, objectives are nothing more or less than desired outcomes. Hence the focus of the case manager on patient outcomes is compatible with an MBO format.

Many newer management tools are based on measurement of outcomes. For example, *benchmarking* implies setting performance targets (usually for aspects of management that lend themselves to easy quantification, such as number of outpatient cases or percentage of charts completed) and comparing these values with prior scores. Comparison may be with one's own prior record, with a competitor's record, or with benchmarking norms established by various professional, managerial, and evaluating or accrediting organizations. The goal in benchmarking is a moving target: always trying to do better in comparison with the prior record.

STRATEGIC MANAGEMENT

Today, most organizations have replaced MBO with strategic management as the primary management method. This is true for freestanding nursing organizations as well as corporations with nursing divisions. Like the resource-driven model of patient care, strategic management starts by assessing the environment—the resources and the immediate situation. From a managerial perspective, assessing the organizational environment involves getting a realistic handle on the internal assets and liabilities of the organization as well as assessing various publics (providers, consumers, payers), other institutions, and legislative and administrative bodies that interface with, or compete with, the organization.

Only after the environment is carefully scanned and assessed are goals selected. They will be goals that can reasonably be taken on, given environmental constraints—goals that optimize the opportunities possible in the milieu. Simplifying the models, one can say that MBO sets out to achieve worthy goals created in the abstract (like goal-driven nursing care), while strategic management (like resource-driven nursing care) picks and chooses where scarce resources will be invested. Typically those investments involve repairing major deficiencies or taking advantage of explicit environmental opportunities. An effective organization is one that makes the best choices for the investments, and intelligent choices depend on making the most accurate assessment of, and the most rapid response to, the immediate situation.

Hence, unlike MBO, strategic management is a resource-driven model of management. Here, immediacy rules, not the long-term future; there is a recognition that the envisioned future may change very rapidly, often because of changes in interacting systems that one cannot control. Not only is the management scheme designed with the environment in mind, but it is made flexible in order to change as the external environment changes. Quick responses are more important than five-year plans. Of necessity, assessment is ongoing rather than periodic. This could be equated with case managers' need to keep up with their patients' outcomes on a daily basis. In strategic management, the outside world impinges on and affects one's plans. The winner is the one who most quickly and accurately interprets and adjusts to (or takes advantage of) the changing situation.

Strategic management may use alternative scenarios, that is, different plans designed to meet different environmental contingencies. The strategic plan recognizes that instability and unpredictability are part of today's world. We live in an era when economic factors are dominant, resources are constrained, and the societal changes that have an impact on health care are not always predictable. In such an era, resource-driven models, from strategic management to managed care, tend to be those best qualified to mesh with the milieu.

Comparing Strategic Management and MBO

To a great degree, resource-driven care and strategic management have replaced goal-driven care and MBO. But this is not to say that one cannot still draw on the best of both systems. The discussion here can be taken to refer to the dominance of the newer models over the older ones.

Strategic management provides for a quick response in a changing world. A typical example is an obstetric department that was feeling the crush of competition from a newer nearby hospital. The solution: a lobster and champagne feast for every client and spouse postdelivery. Although this example is not unique, it points out the fact that the tactics of strategic management may use unique perceptions that are not second nature in nursing. Obviously, lobster and champagne have nothing to do with the quality of care, but they have a lot to do with the client's perceptions and choices.

The traditional MBO planning model has proved of limited value, given the rapid shifts in the environment of today's health care organizations. For example, the imposition of diagnosis related groups (DRGs) caused major upheavals in the long-term plans of many institutions. This was the first prospective plan, reimbursing institutions not for what they did for a patient but on the basis of a projected average cost. As soon as an institution is paid on a prospective basis, that institution starts planning how to use fewer resources to conserve its income. If the prospective payments are already small, then the effectiveness or ineffectiveness of the planning may determine the success or bankruptcy of the providing institution. Managed care and DRGs have taken away the insulation that institutions had under the fee-for-service system.

The imposition of managed care and prices dictated by insurers exerts heavy pressures and brings about a state of continuous upheaval and replanning, in which the interplay of cost factors and quality factors is of prime importance. Consider, for example, a vice president of nursing who is told that a major insurer will no longer reimburse open heart surgery cases at the prior rate. Overnight, the vice president must figure how to reduce nursing costs by 20% for these cases, because a competing institution is willing to provide care at this reduced rate. It does little good when this executive protests that the competitor is providing inferior care.

Mintzberg (1973) identified three different historical strategies for management:

1. *Planning mode:* Characterized by goal setting with systematic and detailed plans for achievement, reliance on rationality and scientific techniques, and anticipatory decision making.
2. *Adaptive mode:* Characterized by reactive and remedial decisions aimed at reducing conflict, ongoing negotiation and adjustment to the environment, and incremental decision making.
3. *Entrepreneurial mode:* Characterized by an active search for new opportunities and proactive leaps forward in the face of uncertainty dominated by a high-risk, high-gain mentality.

If MBO epitomizes the planning mode, then strategic planning can be seen as a modification of both the adaptive mode and the entrepreneurial mode. The entrepreneurial mode is used to take advantage of opportunities, while the adaptive mode corrects weaknesses. Planning ahead is still the aim, but what gets planned depends on the situation, and one must be ready to change plans if circumstances shift. The following assumptions underlie strategic management.

- Management is relational: the major environmental characteristics that have an impact on one's business must be recognized and taken into account in planning.
- The environment may change suddenly and unpredictably, and one must be prepared to change one's plans accordingly—and rapidly.
- Methods and even goals are not fixed but contingent on environmental opportunities.
- Constant surveillance of the environment, including one's competition, is necessary for rapid interpretation and response.

Strategic management is a process that evaluates markets and competition, taking into account the environmental circumstances that are likely to have an impact on the organization. It is a philosophy and method of opportunism, enabling the institution to select goals that accentuate its strengths and market to populations that will benefit from those strengths.

Past missions are explored in light of current organizational realities. New missions are considered pragmatically: What will work to the organization's advantage in these times? This perspective is juxtaposed with an analysis of the potential customers (present or untapped future users of services). The market analysis assesses potential customers in light of environmental factors, primarily economic factors. In most cases the care delivery institution must compete for customers, and its customers include managed care businesses.

Strategic management homes in on major opportunities, isolating trends that will endure and have an impact. It tends to use a broad brush while MBO uses a fine-line pen. Strategic management sets key thrusts for the future, without trying to compose a comprehensive plan for all possible future actions. Strategic management is more flexible than MBO: Commitment to a plan lasts just as long as the plan is effective. When a plan fails, an alternative is quickly put in its place. Failure of a strategic plan is regrettable, but failing to recognize when a plan is not working is a grave managerial error.

The greatest difference between an MBO planning model and strategic management is the different ways in which goals arise. In MBO, all planning begins with goals. In strategic planning, goals are contingent on an analysis of the environment and the potential customers. Decisions involve deciding what the institution is in the best position to produce and market.

Nursing Organizations and Strategic Management

When strategic management uses Mintzberg's entrepreneurial approach, the nurse manager is challenged to develop new revenue streams. To this end, many nurse managers are developing, marketing, and selling new nursing products and services. Along with an entrepreneurial spirit, market survey techniques help the nurse manager determine what nursing products and services can be developed profitably.

For-profit services increase the income of a nursing organization. Customers of these entrepreneurial efforts may be patients, nurses, or other professionals. Nurse-run clinics are one typical example of patient services. Community informational and educational sessions are another source of income. One hospital in an air-polluted environment, for example, developed an ongoing educational series on "Living with Asthma" for the general public.

Many staff development departments market their educational services (e.g., programs preparatory to various credentialing examinations; pharmacy courses) to nurses in their community. Some nursing education departments become self-supporting or even generate revenue with customer-oriented programs.

Nor need traditional programs be the only possible products. If the facility has particular areas of excellence, these specialty can be marketed to produce revenue. For example, an institution with a nationally known cardiovascular program might develop a consultation service or market a short-term nursing internship so that nurses (nationally and internationally) may come to work and learn for a fee.

Nonclinical specialties can be used in this way also. Often organizations with successful case management programs offer consultation services; some market their clinical pathways. If an organization is distinguished in shared governance, materials can be sold or consultation fees can be charged for learning about the program. In programs of this sort, people may come to the facility or experts may go off-site to other institutions.

Internally developed and programmed learning texts and videotapes, or various manuals (patient education, clinical pathways, nursing procedures), are all products being created and marketed to generate revenue. With an entrepreneurial marketing orientation, nursing develops many revenue generating products.

Nor need products be limited to nurse clients. Some staff development programs, for example, are selling programs required for relicensure (e.g., education regarding child abuse education and infection control) to practitioners from all professions. Outside of traditional acute care, nurses are forming their own corporations and companies for various health care services. They market well-health programs to industry, alternative-site care to ill and convalescent customers, and life enhancement and recovery programs to the growing health-conscious public.

Strategic management opens new possibilities for nurses in old and new settings, established and new businesses. In many cases, nurses are competing successfully with physicians and other providers, offering similar services at competitive prices.

EDUCATIONAL IMPLICATIONS

The faculty member must understand the radical changes in the times and temperament that dominate health care today. This is the world that the student will enter upon graduation: fast-paced, competitive, and business-oriented. The world is changing fast, and the student who does not recognize the nature of the work world will be at a distinct disadvantage. Clinical education alone is no longer adequate. It does no good to know individual trees if you cannot find your way through the forest.

The faculty member can help prepare students for today's challenging health care context by giving them practice in dealing with clinical and administrative problems encountered in the clinical facility. Students can be encouraged to apply and compare goal-driven MBO and resource-driven strategic management approaches.

Much of today's nursing education involves the addition of new process skills to a curriculum that once was content-driven. Students who have some successes—for example, in applying strategic management techniques—will be better prepared for the world of work.

SUMMARY

Running a nursing organization may be streamlined if the processes of nursing administration and the processes of care management are similar. This goal can be achieved by matching goal-driven models or linking resource-driven models. Like total patient care (or care by nursing diagnosis and the nursing care plan), management by objective is a goal-driven administrative model. Like care delivery that starts with an assessment of clinical resources for care (prioritized care), strategic management is a resource-driven model.

Any organization will probably use aspects from both models, but one will be dominant. In today's environment, the rest of the facility is more likely to be using resource-driven models of management. If the nursing department wishes to be compatible with today's management formats, it will need to adopt resource-driven care and nursing management models that reflect strategic planning. Such models allow for adapting to the changing environment and encourage the department to take advantage of entrepreneurial opportunities that may come its way.

REFERENCES

Barnum, B. S. (1998). *Nursing theory: Analysis, application, evaluation* (5th ed.). Philadelphia: Lippincott.
Barnum, B. S., & Kerfoot, K. M. (1995). *The nurse as executive* (4th ed.). Gaithersburg, MD: Aspen.
Mintzberg, H. (1973). Strategy-making in three modes. *California Management Review, 16*(2): 44–53.

TEST YOUR UNDERSTANDING

Multiple-Choice

Select the one *best* answer.

1. *In what way is benchmarking similar to management by objectives? Both:*
   a. Are new methods of management.
   b. Require lots of quantitative data.
   c. Are goal-driven systems.
   d. Are resource-driven systems.

2. *Compared with MBO, what is the time frame for strategic planning?*
   a. Strategic planning is longer-term.
   b. Strategic planning has no time frame whatsoever.
   c. Strategic planning is shorter-term.
   d. Strategic planning does not set endpoints in time.

3. *Why have we moved to shorter-term planning models?*
   a. The future is difficult because of cost containment.
   b. Resources to ensure that long-term plans will be funded are lacking.
   c. There is little time for long-term planning.
   d. The distant future cannot be predicted with any accuracy.

4. *Which of the following is a managerial* flaw *under strategic planning?*
   a. Miscalculating the upcoming future scenario.
   b. Sticking to a strategic plan that no longer seems to be working.
   c. Making a bold plan that involves some risks.
   d. Creating plans with broad directives rather than with finite details.

Discussion of Answers

1. a. Although benchmarking is new, at least in popularity, MBO is a traditional method.
   b. While both systems may use quantitative data, this hardly characterizes their similarity. Indeed, some MBO goals may be "soft," rather than amenable to a numerical interpretation.
   c. This is the correct answer.
   d. These systems are not resource-driven.

2. a. MBO sets long-term plans; strategic planning seldom does.
   b. Objectives set without an endpoint in mind could never be evaluated.
   c. This is the correct answer.
   d. Any objective needs an endpoint, even if it is close in time.

3. a. The fact that a future may be difficult does not mean that it cannot be planned for.
   b. One could always make plans fit the resources, if that were the issue.
   c. Time needed to do planning has nothing to do with timing factors within the planning.
   d. This is the correct answer.

4. a. Anyone can miscalculate when the future is fluid, even with the best of plans.
   b. This is the correct answer.
   c. High risks with a potential for big gains are a part of strategic planning.
   d. Strategic plans seldom are as detailed as the old MBO plans.

8

School and Societal Environments

Managed care affects many aspects of nursing education, both directly and indirectly. In this chapter, we will examine the relationship of nursing education to society at large and to health care delivery institutions. Chapter 9 will examine nursing as an educational unit of a college or university, as well as changes in nursing programs, alterations in the role of the faculty, and resultant methods of teacher-student interface. The forces that have created managed care in care delivery settings have had a similar impact on educational institutions at large and on the nursing departments within them. Simply put, resource-driven management has invaded the university and college setting. Under this new pressure, nursing departments have their own vulnerabilities and opportunities.

NURSING EDUCATION AND SOCIETY AT LARGE

As we have seen in earlier chapters, managed care was a response to a public outcry over the high cost of health care. Care delivery was the first sector to come under close scrutiny regarding costs, but the principle was soon applied to other sectors of society, including education. The questions raised were similar: What are we getting for our education dollar? What are the educational products? Could we have an equal or better product for the same cost? In part, these questions were raised because the costs of education, like the costs of health care, had continued to escalate. A major concern was the fact that tuition had grown by leaps and bounds, threatening to put unsubsidized collegiate education out of reach of the middle class. Hence, education, once a relatively insular social institution, was moved into the present era of cost containment.

All educational programs that dealt with preparing health care workers found themselves exposed to two sources of pressure: (1) the demands for cost savings that were being applied to the health care industry in particular, and (2) the growing demand for cost savings in education. The demands on health care settings had a trickle-down effect on education, for various reasons which we will explore.

Major changes in practice had a significant impact on nursing education: (1) a decreased demand for and, at least until recently, fewer employment opportunities for registered nurses; (2) a need for effective education of unlicensed assistive personnel; (3) the *de facto* effect that certain nursing roles became "winner" or "losers" in the new delivery system. The existence of managed care changed the nature of the workforce; and when the nature of the workforce changed, its educational needs also changed, as did opportunities and vulnerabilities in nursing education.

Less Demand for Registered Nurses in the Workforce

One of the greatest changes affecting nursing education in the 1990s was the fact that virtually overnight nursing went from a seller's to a buyer's market. A decade earlier, persons entering nursing assumed that, upon graduation from any type of program, they could pick and choose among job offers. Instead, graduates of many nursing programs faced up to a year or more of searching to find any nursing position and longer to locate a preferred position.

The effect was to decrease the attractiveness of nursing as a career, and subsequently to decrease applications to nursing schools for beginning RN preparation. Unfortunately, as this societal change took place, few nursing organizations or schools asked the obvious question: If there is less demand for nurses in the workforce, should we still try to prepare the same numbers? Instead, most schools simply stuck to business as usual. Systems thinking was not applied to the distribution problems. The laws of supply and demand were fought tooth and nail. Indeed, this same separation of the schooling function from the working function had been seen earlier when schools and education organizations banded together in a public advertising campaign to increase applications. This method had been successful for its duration, despite its defiance of what was happening in the hiring world.

Faculties everywhere, vulnerable to job threats if their student numbers shrank, pressed to maintain or increase their admissions. Even when the inescapable trend of retrenchment became obvious, few schools voluntarily closed. Instead, the typical school competed for the requisite students. The decrease in applicants sent schools scrambling to meet their quotas and caused them to become customer-oriented in the pursuit of, and competition for, students. Programs that once had created hurdles to admission, attendance, or completion suddenly discovered that they could make consumer-friendly adaptations in order to attract and keep students.

Faculties across the nation realized that to survive, they had to widen their nets; but increased recruitment efforts aimed at high school seniors proved difficult. Unfortunately, many faculties responded by lowering their admissions standards. Schools that had previously sought honor-roll students began to accept the C-average student. Across the nation one could see a general decline in standards—ironically, just at a time when graduating nurses would need even more acumen to work effectively and survive in the system.

Wooing mature people who desired a second career was a more effective strategy for many schools, especially as other fields went through their own retrenchments. Ultimately, the entry of second-career students was narrowed by the increasing journalistic focus on nurses' being laid off and unable to find jobs.

Whatever the individual efforts of each school, for perhaps the first time many faculties began to look at education as a business. The era of competitive marketing that had earlier invaded health care delivery descended on nursing education as well.

As nursing schools became more skilled at operating as businesses, they learned the advantage of creating special niches and meeting marketplace demands. Numerous contemporary studies focused faculties' attention on the actual nursing needs required in the changing system. Perhaps the most influential of these was the Pew Commission report (1995), which recommended a 20% reduction in training programs for nurses, indicating that remaining programs needed to be redirected toward 4-year and, particularly, advanced practice.

Many collegiate faculties got the message and focused on producing more advanced practitioners. Schools shifted their numbers toward increased graduate students, concurrently decreasing the number of beginning students, with some schools actually closing their first-level programs. Other schools reduced their total numbers in response to the societal message, but often the game afoot was to shift the emphasis of programs rather than to decrease the total size of the student body.

In general, nursing schools ignored the societal demand for fewer nurses, putting their own survival first. It is difficult to blame them, because the environment created in the nation was one of competition, designed to let the weaker fish be swallowed by the stronger ones. If this situation continues, with the competition becoming more fierce, we will probably see more schools closing.

At present, however, there appears to be a correction of the situation, with an increased demand for RNs in the marketplace in some locations.

Whether this turns out to be a steady trend or simply a small blip in the downward market demand remains to be seen. Whatever the next trend, nursing education has received a lesson in how closely it is tied to the demands of the marketplace. The link is unlikely ever to be ignored again.

Educational Needs of Unlicensed Assistive Personnel

In the recent shrinkage, one way that schools of nursing could prolong or cushion their survival was to diversify, that is, to find new tasks for the faculty to do or new groups for the faculty to teach. In respect to the latter strategy, there was a whole new population with educational needs: unlicensed assistive personnel (UAPs), whose jobs were created to assist the decreasing numbers of RNs. As complaints concerning unprepared UAPs grew, opportunities for schools to take over education contracts also grew. Some schools found themselves in competition for UAP education assignments with internal departments of nursing education in service organizations. Often these departments were involved in their own struggle against retrenchment. New and diverse liaisons were formed between collegiate nursing educators and educators in the service sector.

Although some schools (often community colleges) got into UAP education, other schools, particularly universities and prestigious collegiate programs, declined to take on the education of subordinate personnel.

Nevertheless, for some schools a move into education of UAPs represented a first venture into meeting marketplace needs for the sake of keeping a program solvent. As happened in care delivery, the education faculty was shifting toward strategic management, in which the nature of the environment is assessed and programs are planned accordingly.

Winning and Losing Nursing Roles

In the changing health care scene, some nursing roles gained advantages while other roles lost status. It was difficult, for example, for nursing executives to justify keeping those clinical nurse specialists (CNSs) whose assignments were simply to do what regular staff nurses did, only better. Such staff CNS positions frequently were the first to go when nurse executives were trying to retain as many positions as possible under stringent budget cuts.

On the other hand, nurse practitioner roles that could save money by replacing more expensive physician roles were retained and expanded. Schools of nursing responded by converting clinical specialist programs to practitioner programs or by creating new programs in which working clinical specialists could learn the added skills that would qualify them for licensing as practitioners. Virtually overnight, practitioner preparation became the way a nursing program could deal with the problem of dwindling students. Practitioner education was a winning game, and many schools rushed to join the bandwagon. The number of schools presently preparing practitioners now threatens to create an oversupply in this category as well. Indeed, in some large cities, practitioners already are having difficulty finding positions.

Another solution used by some schools was to create programs for preparation in a new role in managed care: nursing case manager. This role demanded nurses who could demonstrate special skills: an orientation toward patient outcomes along with exquisite assessment skills and familiarity with case management mapping. While some schools successfully established programs of case management, on the whole these have not been as successful as the programs of practitioner education, simply because not every nurse wants to stake his or her future on the continuance of managed care as a delivery format.

Nevertheless, schools have responded to the marketplace. The motivation for the response, unique in the history of nursing education, may have been self-serving, but educators had learned how to respond to marketplace demands when they must.

RELATIONSHIP OF NURSING EDUCATION TO PRACTICE INSTITUTIONS

Faculty relationships with practice organizations have become integral and integrated because the fate of education is now perceived as affected by what happens in practice. This attitude is in contrast to the erstwhile patrician notion on the part of many educators that education would call the tune and set the future path for practice. The number of interfaces between practice and education had already grown in the years shortly before case management came on the scene, partly because each side (practice and education) had come to understand that it had much to gain from a partnership. The changes that were under way when managed care appeared had to do with joint practice-education roles, using practice nurses as preceptors, extending faculty appointments to certain practitioners, and other exchange measures then seen as innovative.

Managed care, however, created an environment where each side took a more critical view of what it had to gain and lose in these new relationships. The service agencies, which had typically gotten lesser benefits from these deals, quickly turned the tables. The first criterion by which deals were now assessed in a practice institution involved cost, not prior professional values. Gone, for example, was one old value—the idea that practicing nurses had an obligation to bring along the next generation of nursing students. Now the motto was: only if it pays.

The "fair exchange" principle still offers something for everyone, and today exchanges can be seen that include but are not limited to these: (1) faculty appointments for clinicians in exchange for preceptorships; (2) faculty-run continuing education programs in exchange for clinical placements for students; (3) faculty assistance with research projects that are going on in the practice setting; (4) competition, cooperation, or both among various schools for favored clinical experience hours; and (5) joint faculty-service nursing clinics or centers.

Several changes within the last decade have made reciprocal exchanges easier. First, there are now many nurse clinicians with the requisite academic credentials for university and college faculty appointments. These nurses range from vice presidents of nursing to incumbents in other supervisory nursing layers, often down to head nurses.

Interchanges between practice and education often involve altered roles. These roles vary from place to place and may be found on every level, from the clinical staff nurse who has a caseload of students as well as a caseload of patients, all the way up to the nursing vice president who is also a dean. Sometimes, as in the latter example, the roles are administrative in both settings; sometimes they are not. For example, a dean might carry a caseload of patients in a private practice. The danger in an era of reduced resources is that these mixed roles may make excessive demands on the incumbent, each portion demanding nearly a full-time commitment.

Nevertheless, it is not only a philosophic commitment to unity between education and practice that brings such roles into existence; in many cases, it is cost-effectiveness. For example, costs may be reduced by having one executive over service and education within a single parent institution. Frequently now, one sees a deanship of a school of nursing and a vice presidency of the nursing division of the associated university hospital held by one incumbent. Of course, there is some professional vulnerability in this model; sometimes these executive nursing positions are eliminated, leaving a subordinate manager in each component in charge, often reporting one level lower in the organizational chain of command.

Another reason that joint roles are popular is the shift in earning power between practice and education. The turnaround in the last decade has been dramatic, with service salaries not only equaling, but commonly surpassing, faculty rates. In other words, it may well be financially worth a faculty member's time to have a concomitant practice role.

One practice that got caught in the press of economics is the use of clinical preceptors to educate students. A decade or more ago, many nursing schools put into place practice preceptorships whereby qualified practitioners provided the main clinical supervision for one or more students, the faculty member serving primarily to set up the relationships, negotiate objectives among parties, agree to oral or written learning contracts, monitor ongoing relationships, and consult with the preceptor to arrive at a student's grade.

This was—and still is in some places—an excellent design because it provides the role modeling that is difficult when a student learns primarily from a faculty member. After all, the student is learning to be in practice, not learning to be a faculty member. It makes more sense for the closest mentor to demonstrate the role to which the student aspires. Role inculcation is certainly speeded up with this model.

A problem with cost controls arises under managed care, however. Under the pressures of resource-driven delivery, practice preceptors no longer have the extra time required to teach and monitor students properly. Often the preceptor withdraws from the relationship. Nor is withdrawal only on the part of individual preceptors. Many organizations, conscious of the time constraints on their employees, have refused to ratify these practicum models. Once, having students on a unit was perceived as increasing the staff available for service; now students are seen as one more burden. Indeed, some service organizations are demanding financial compensation from schools of nursing for precepting students.

This altered perception has thrust the responsibility for clinical education back on the faculty. As with many aspects of a cost-conscious environment, there is no easy answer. Sometimes increasing the benefit for the service institution will produce an agreement to continue the preceptor model. For example, providing faculty appointments for clinical preceptors or giving free continuing education classes for the service institution may be a trading chip. Everyone has learned to play the resource-driven game, and faculties cannot expect to get something for nothing these days.

SUMMARY

How a nursing program operates has become very much a result of pressures from its environment. The environment includes aspects of change within the entire society and in the world of health care delivery. The change involves demands for cost-effective education that does not eat up care delivery resources. Of necessity, education has had to respond to these environmental demands. Hence, resource-driven management is becoming the way in which academe is managed as well as the pattern in service.

Further, as more faculty members combine practice and education functions in a single job, education gains more people with personal experience in the managed care system. The growth of practitioner models in education has also fostered an intake of faculty members who have prior experience with managed care in the service sector.

REFERENCES

Pew Health Professions Commission. (1995). *Critical challenges: Revitalizing the health professions for the twenty-first century.* San Francisco, CA: Author.

TEST YOUR UNDERSTANDING

Multiple-Choice
Select the one *best* answer.

1. *What was the typical response by schools to decreased demands for practicing nurses?*
   a. To decrease their student admissions.
   b. To attempt to change the practice situation.
   c. To market their programs to new potential groups of students.

2. *Which of the following tactics was* least *effective in attracting students to nursing programs?*
   a. Extensive advertising through the public media.
   b. Renewed efforts to attract high school seniors.
   c. Appeals to people seeking a second career.

3. *What was the* chief *factor that changed the relationship of the school of nursing to the home, college, or practice setting?*
   a. Demands for increased productivity on the part of practice.
   b. The fact that practice personnel now held more advanced degrees.
   c. The fact that schools began using more community settings.

4. *Which of the following roles lost status under managed care?*
   a. Clinical specialist.
   b. Nurse practitioner.
   c. Case manager.

5. *Why have many clinical staff nurses refused to become preceptors for student nurses?*
   a. Students are less intelligent than they once were, making the preceptor's job more difficult.
   b. Staff nurses lack the necessary time to invest in students.
   c. Staff nurses make more money if they stick to practice tasks.

Discussion of Answers

1. a. Most schools did not voluntarily decrease admissions.
   b. Schools did not concern themselves with the nuances of managed care; indeed, many failed to understand the changes under way.
   c. This is the correct answer.

2. a. Advertising was extremely successful in generating interest in nursing programs through a public media campaign.
   b. This is the correct answer.
   c. Many schools depended on this strategy, designing their programs to cater to this market.

3. a. This is the correct answer.
   b. This is true, but it was not the greatest influence on changing relationships.
   c. This is true, but it was not the greatest influence on changing relationships.

4. a. This is the correct answer.
   b. Under managed care, nurse practitioners gained because they could replace more costly physicians.
   c. The case manager is a very powerful role because it mediates outcomes, usually for other professions as well as nursing.

5. a. Students' intelligence is not the major factor in this decision.
   b. This is the correct answer.
   c. Salaries are seldom greater because one *refuses* to mentor students.

9

The Nursing Department in the College or University

Often nursing faculties and their leadership lack a clear perception of where nursing stands in the university or college at large. In part, this is due to a narrowed and insular focus on nursing alone. There are many reasons why nursing faculties have long been focused inward, and that focus has helped nursing move toward professional maturity. However, in an era when the environment is the controlling factor, an inward focus makes nursing vulnerable and must be abandoned.

Hence, the first task of a faculty is to see how others in the institution see the nursing department or school. The term *nursing department* will be used generically in this chapter to indicate the full range of educational units: a college of nursing, a school of nursing, a department, a program of nursing. Similarly, the term *college* will cover the range of schools from a community college to a college to a university. Many presidents of colleges (as well as their governing boards) see nursing as a worthy but middle-class endeavor not likely to bring the institution much prestige. Nursing graduates—not likely to make a fortune, not apt to give the institution a substantial endowment—are seen as a gift to the community, but not as a great payoff for the college or university itself.

From the perspective of most other departments, the nursing program may be next to invisible; again, this is a result of nursing's inward focus. Only when there is a serious problem with nursing services in a community will academic colleagues take notice of what is happening in the nursing program. In some eras, not being noticed can be a good thing; but in the present situation, nursing is more often noticed for its failures than its successes.

NURSING DEPARTMENTS UNDER FIRE

Like care delivery facilities, educational institutions are facing an era of fiscal retrenchment. Such retrenchment causes an increase in internal competition for resources. In this competition, a nursing department may be especially vulnerable. Often a nursing program requires (or its faculty thinks it requires) more resources than other departments. For example, nursing faculties claim that their clinical supervision requires a greater faculty-student ratio than the social work department or the program in dance arts. If the need for more resources is genuine, and if other departments have better established research programs or are perceived as more prestigious (for example, those same departments of social work and dance), then the department of nursing is setting itself up as a target for elimination when the institution retrenches.

Every few months, most nursing leaders receive desperate calls or letters asking them to write to one or another college president asking that he or she reconsider a planned elimination of a nursing program. Some of these mass write-in campaigns are successful; most are not. College presidents do not mark for elimination programs that can mount serious objections. Nor do they target for elimination programs that contribute substantially to the institution's financial welfare. Whether we view it as natural or nasty, the best targets for retrenchment are: (1) departments requiring high input of resources (e.g., a high ratio of faculty to students), (2) departments seen as already weak and vulnerable (e.g., with no important political allies), and (3) departments that bring little to the institution from a financial perspective (e.g., those who bring only tuition income and few big donors). Often nursing departments meet all these criteria.

In this era, nursing departments are challenged to be politically savvy, clever, and not costly. Often the threat of closure is what makes a department of nursing suddenly adopt a business orientation, and this may involve applying a resource-driven model to educational management. Even the most secure of nursing departments cannot forget that it is in internal competition with all the other departments of the college or university for scarce resources.

Many nursing programs now face the same sort of demand for economy of resources that the care delivery sector faced earlier. The principles, if not the programs, of managed care have invaded academe, and failure to understand that may make a program vulnerable to loss of resources or even to elimination.

STRATEGIC PLANNING FOR NURSING DEPARTMENTS

When a nursing department systematically examines its program, what questions need to be asked from a business orientation. More specifically, what questions arise in applying a resource-driven model? The questions listed here would not surprise any business, but not all faculties think to ask them.

1. What is our purpose? Why do we exist? What societal benefits do we provide? What benefits do we bring to the college or university?
2. What are our products? What characterizes our graduates? Are there any products apart from our graduates? For example, to what valuable research do we contribute? What important patient and community services do we provide? (The elements that constitute "products" may vary from school to school, depending on the program's activities.)
3. Who is our competition? Who provides similar services or products? How do we differentiate ourselves from our competitors? What is our added value beyond that of the competitors? Can the community support two or more similar programs?
4. Should we exist? (The answer to this question is derived from the answers to the prior questions.)
5. If we should exist, what strategies should we take to survive and thrive?

What Is Our Purpose?

CONSIDERING THE PURPOSE

Peculiarly, few programs of nursing education ever ask the first questions concerning one's reason for being: What is our purpose? Why do we exist? What societal benefits do we provide? What benefits do we bring to the college or university? If these questions arise, it is often because the continued existence of a program is threatened. When this occurs, it may be too late to consider these goal-oriented questions in an orderly fashion.

Often the faculty of a department of nursing gives little thought to its purpose. From a societal perspective, the department usually has served a historical function of supplying needed professionals for the local community. Today, that purpose may have evaporated in the wake of the restructuring and downsizing that have swept over health care, beginning in acute care and spreading to alternative care settings.

The belief has been that displaced nurses will find new positions in community care delivery systems and in home care. Yet realistically, the principle of cost-efficiency (including lean hiring policies) has spread down-ward, along with the shift of patients to alternative facilities. Further, what-ever portion of the health care dollar goes into preventive care under the managed care system is designed to prevent more costly (and more staff-intensive) acute care. While it is too soon to predict how many nurses will be required when the system is totally reconstituted, it is likely that there will be an overall adjustment downward from the number employed before managed care. Certainly this trend has been felt in big cities, where some graduates search for up to a year for a job—any job, not their preferred job.

Alternatively, there may be periods of radical shifts in nursing demand. Indeed, at the moment, we seem to have a pendulum shift toward the hir-ing of more nurses. Possibly, the impetus has been the recent criticism of several major care delivery systems because of serious failures in nursing care, due in turn to understaffing. In any case, the community service that once justified a nursing department's existence may be on shaky ground at the moment.

If one believes the Pew Health Professions Commission (1995), we will need a 20% reduction in our training capacity for nurses, but seldom does a faculty think that *its* department should be one to close. If we allow each department the right to compete for survival, we must recognize that pre-dictions of decreased societal need weaken a nursing department's power within the local college or university community. Such predictions give a president who wishes to eliminate a department of nursing a strong weapon.

What does the president know of the nursing department's purpose? How critical is the department in his or her perception? What has been done by the nursing faculty to shape the president's perceptions? Strategic management principles focus on marketing, and this strategy should also be applied within the college. The president, his or her administration, the governing board, and other academic departments are important targets for marketing efforts by the nursing department.

CREATING NEEDS

If one grants a department the right to compete for survival irrespective of the society's projected need for manpower, then one does not truly "begin at the beginning" in planning a program of nursing education. Instead of the logical order (in which a societal need gives impetus to the creation of a program), we have an existing program looking for a reason to continue. Self-interest may lead a nursing program to search out a special niche or even to create a "need" that was not perceived previously in the communi-ty. This situation is far from new; many business enterprises search for new reasons to exist when old reasons grow obsolete. Indeed, a spectacularly successful business may not only create a unique product but engender a desire for that product in the marketplace.

In earlier chapters, we saw that strategic planning is a management tool compatible with a resource-driven model of care, such as managed care. The same model applied to a program of nursing education is useful in determining *mission* and *purpose*—the formal terms applied in academe to the overarching goal and the broad underlying objective or objectives. Mission and purpose are not selected in isolation. Indeed, before determining its own mission, a nursing department should be aware of the college's mission. Typically, this mission has been assigned in the school's charter. Whatever the nursing unit determines to do, it must be in accord with that institutional mission. Indeed, the department that is perceived as contributing directly to achievement of the college's central mission will be perceived as a valuable showpiece by the administration.

Before determining where one is headed (selecting goals that contribute to college and departmental mission), the department should assess its societal and college environments. The college environment includes the administration, other units and departments, the political environment, alumni, accreditation status and activities, and the place of this institution in the intercollegiate world.

The societal environment is complex and extensive, for it involves every community interacting with the college and the nursing department. A nursing department in a large city with an international student body and a small department in a sparsely populated region of the country might identify vastly different environments as pertinent. In each case, though, the health care environment is only one part of a total societal environment.

The nursing department's mission and purpose are likely to emerge from negotiation between societal needs (local, national, and, if appropriate, international) and the unique circumstances of the college and nursing department. The departmental purpose should have some benefit for all of these constituencies. It should also be influenced by productive interchange with the practice environment, because that element is important in providing clinical learning experiences.

What Are Our Products?

After assessing the relevant environments and setting a mission and a purpose, the department is ready to determine what sort of products could achieve the goals. Products bring the mission to life. Most nursing departments view their graduates as their most important product. Yet what characterizes one's graduates can be determined on various levels, from the legal-technical perspective (e.g., we will produce baccalaureate and graduate nurses with advanced clinical and technological expertise) to the most esoteric characteristics (e.g., what specific personal values our graduates will hold).

What constitutes a product may vary from department to department depending on the type (or types) of nurses in demand in the assessed environments. The successful faculty targets a unique niche in the marketplace, one it feels best equipped to supply. Because graduates are the most important products of a nursing education program, one must ask whether there is a realistic need for the program's present graduates. If not, the department may be able to identify types of nurses needed by the community (or communities) it serves. If the department is to remain viable, it must to find or create a demand niche.

Many departments enhance their security by creating products above and beyond their graduates. For example, some departments are known for their contributions to the profession—for instance, through valuable research programs. Others provide valuable patient and community services which often enhance relations between the college and the community. Nurse-run clinics are one popular example in this category.

Additionally, the department must assess what it contributes directly to the parent college. Is the nursing faculty active on important out-of-department committees and task forces? Does it provide students for courses that other departments wish to fill? An insular nursing program with few identified exchanges with other programs is vulnerable. Sometimes important products that contribute to the life and welfare of a college are not acknowledged until they are made evident by the nursing department, often in quantitative terms. Again, marketing oneself is essential. Newsletters or journals from the nursing department may partially fill this purpose.

Alumni are another important, if sometimes unrecognized, product. Alumni groups and individuals should be courted. Alumni should be financial supporters of the department and its programs, but this doesn't happen without effort. The nursing department must establish channels for continued reinvolvement by alumni. A dean can have no worse enemy than a disaffected alumni group. When there are major changes in any programs, soliciting the approval and support of alumni is a critical strategy.

Who Is Our Competition?

Just as products cannot be selected in a vacuum, a decision concerning products should not be finalized without considering the third set of questions: Who is our competition? Who provides similar services or products? How can we differentiate ourselves from our competitors? What is our added value beyond that of the competitors? How many programs can the community support, for example, in terms of future jobs and present locations for clinical experiences?

The department must assess its educational rivals. What other nursing departments in the area are perceived as vying for the same selected niche or niches? If a competitor is better equipped to service a niche, the department might need to reassess and find another focus. Alternatively, the department might decide how it could interest a different (new) population of potential students, or how it might attract students away from the competition.

If a department has no competitors, it is fortunate. Next best is having a unique niche for which others are ill prepared to compete, or a product that offers distinct advantages over the competitors' products. Convenient time schedules for students, cost advantages, and a sterling reputation are illustrations. One must have something to market. To distinguish oneself from the competition requires a consumer orientation. What do today's students look for in selecting a program?

It pays to be the first to come up with products other than students, such as nurse-run clinics or continuing education programs. Unfortunately, a successful idea is quickly copied, and one may be rest assured that last year's blue-ribbon product will soon be surrounded by numerous "me too" packages from the competition. What inevitably happens is that the community is soon oversaturated, and the products begin to lose money for everyone. Finding new, competitive products is the name of the game.

Should We Exist?

One sees in education today the same sort of consortia and mergers that earlier characterized the practice environment. Indeed, some of the more interesting linkages include both practice and educational institutions. Such linkages may enhance security for all parties. Hence, competition is not the only possible approach to growth and survival. Cooperation among disparate departments and practice organizations has created strong networks and interesting formal or informal mergers. Departments have aligned themselves in horizontal networks (e.g., shared resources among graduate nursing programs) and in vertical networks (e.g., educational "articulated ladders" among various associate, baccalaureate, and graduate programs). Cooperation may offer something for everyone.

A department needs to justify its existence. When a department is unable to satisfy its various constituencies or produce a satisfactory and needed product, it must consider whether it should continue. It is better that the faculty reach a closure decision before "higher-ups" do, so that there is time for an orderly dismantling of a program.

Strategies for Survival

When a department believes it should continue, it still must consider what strategies and tactics to use in a resource-driven institution. Most of those strategies involve running education like a business, and that threatens some of the longest-held values of the educational community. Leisurely and democratic deliberation by the faculty is one of the first values to be sacrificed when the speed of decisions may determine whether or not a department will be able to capture a market or receive some other timely benefit. Tenure also is being shed by many schools, in an effort to enhance the quality of their products, especially where budgets no longer have enough slack to support minimal contributors.

Consider this realistic assessment of a program's likelihood of survival. The author is a dean of a private school of nursing:

> It is reasonable to ask whether any private schools of medicine or nursing will remain open after the year 2000 because of their expense. The most viable model for survival of these schools requires the generation of new ideas and new sources of revenue, such as practice revenue, to fuel the research and teaching engines. (Conway-Welch, 1996, p. 288)

Nursing departments are learning to apply cost-benefit and cost-effectiveness models that are already being used in the service sector.

NETWORKING

One of the strategies used today by vulnerable nursing departments is to become less insular. Often this involves organizing joint courses with other disciplines such as medicine, dentistry, and social work. Or it may involve joint work with a business school, with a school of public health, or even with disciplines and departments that have a less obvious connection to nursing. Nursing departments have abandoned their prior prejudice that students must get their required course content taken in other departments reinterpreted in the nursing department. Now faculties credit nursing students with being able to translate and apply material learned in other parts of the college. Such expanded vision serves students well, while enabling the nursing department to conserve its shrinking resources and enhance its value to other departments.

Increased participation in the larger college community provides a network of relations and colleagues that may support a vulnerable nursing department in the future. Simply put, it is more difficult to excise a nursing program with broad networks and intercollegiate commitments than it is to excise an insular program. Nor is protection the only advantage of an integrated approach; nursing students benefit greatly from the broader horizons they acquire from mixing with others students in other departments.

GIFTS TO THE COLLEGE

Gifts to the college come in many forms, chief among them high visibility, prestige, and income. Nursing departments should examine all options.

Showcasing of special products has become an expectation for any nursing dean who hopes to remain long in the position. Showcase products or events ensure a long tenure for a department. Showcase products are those that have publicity appeal, bring in funds, or in some other way make the department and the college both look good. Often, nursing departments are involved with events or provide services that could be showcased for the larger college and the local community with just a little publicity or a slight shift in orientation. The showcase product must be one easily explainable to larger interested publics. For example, the nursing department in one university created a program for teenage community opinion leaders, teaching them how to influence their peers concerning violence, AIDS, and teenage pregnancy. Part of the program consisted of improving the teenagers' communication skills through learning to speak to groups via various media. In one assignment the teenagers created a television drama, showing themselves "in action" with other young people. This created an easily marketable, ready-made clip picked up by local television stations, reflecting well on town-gown relations for the whole university.

Another gift to the home institution is fund-raising. Even if those funds are dedicated to the nursing department, they probably replace other funds the college would otherwise have to supply. Development work (as fund-raising is sometimes called) has assumed the level of big business, with the dean's role, more than ever, involving cultivating relationships with actual or potential donors. Some nursing departments additionally use a public relations firm as a vehicle for creating visibility, building new publics, and impressing donors.

OTHER STRATEGIES

Other strategies for survival include reasonable control over important indicators of fiscal performance such as student-faculty ratios, adequate enrollment, and an adequate number of graduates. The ability to attract grants is also important, as is a national or even an international reputation. Some of these strategies will be discussed in subsequent chapters.

SUMMARY

The nursing faculty must be cognizant of the department's real and perceived standing among its peer departments and divisions within the college. Maintaining the right appearance can be very important. This is an era when a nursing program will benefit from being solidly within the web of the college instead of isolating itself and its students. One must strategically plan to make others aware of the contributions of the nursing department to the college and to the community at large.

REFERENCES

Conway-Welch, C. (1996). Who is tomorrow's nurse and where will tomorrow's nurse be educated? *Nursing and Health Care: Perspectives on Community, 17*(6): 286–290.
Pew Health Professions Commission. (1995). *Critical challenges: Revitalizing the health professions for the twenty-first century.* San Francisco, CA: Author.

TEST YOUR UNDERSTANDING

Multiple-Choice

Select the one *best* answer.

1. *Which description characterizes today's relationship between a college and its department of nursing?*
   a. The two are adversarial, making the nursing department a target for retrenchment.
   b. The relationship is paternal; the college will decide what resources it gives to the nursing department.
   c. A reciprocal relationship is required in which the department contributes to the college as well as vice versa.

2. *What is the relationship of the nursing department's mission to the college's mission?*
   a. They are identical.
   b. The nursing department's mission should advance the college's mission.
   c. No relationship between the two goal statements is required.
   d. The nursing division does not need to have a mission, but the college does.

3. *Why is tenure disappearing from many campuses?*
   a. Resource reduction prevents retention of members on a principle that is indifferent to cost.
   b. Faculty members' free speech is no longer protected by tenure, so it has become obsolete.
   c. Faculties no longer support the principle of tenure.

4. *Why is the continuation of nursing departments threatened today in many colleges?*
   a. Nursing has little prestige.
   b. Nurses are oversupplied in the nation.
   c. Nursing programs require major revamping.
   d. Nursing programs are often not cost-effective.

Discussion of Answers

1. a. Although a nursing department may become a target for retrenchment, that fact is usually not based on an adversarial relationship with the college.
   b. This is the old model, which is now undergoing a change.
   c. This is the correct answer.

2. a. The two missions need not be identical.
   b. This is the correct answer.
   c. They should be related at least to the extent that they are mutually compatible.
   d. Without a mission, the nursing department will have no sense of direction.

3. a. This is the correct answer.
   b. The change in tenure policies has nothing to do with free speech.
   c. While some faculties see tenure as "old fashioned," few voluntarily give up a protective right.

4. a. Nursing may or may not have prestige in a given community or college, but this is seldom the reason for removing an extant program.
   b. Few colleges drop programs as a direct response to the nation's need, even though oversupply may become an indirect factor.
   c. Nursing programs may need revamping, but this is seldom a reason for eliminating them.
   d. This is the correct answer.

10

The Nursing Program:
Looking Inward

Although a nursing department needs to look outward, to see its place in the college and in the community at large, it must also look inward. The curriculum for each nursing program needs to be reviewed in light of today's environmental pressures. Indeed, old programs may need to be exchanged for entirely new ones. In addition to making decisions about the curriculum, faculties need to understand how their roles have undergone change as a result of the same environmental and economic pressures.

THE NURSING PROGRAM OF STUDIES

Determining internal programs of study is of major importance to a nursing education department. Two essential areas for decisions involve: (1) which programs to offer, and (2) the content of those programs. Both decisions may be critical to the welfare of a nursing program.

Which Programs to Offer

In the past, most nursing departments made the same decision concerning what programs would be offered; that is (with exception of the associate degree departments, which will not be considered here), they all had a bachelor's program and then, if possible, added a master's program. Those who could go farther added the doctoral program. The dominant notion was an ascending hierarchy of programs, with the doctoral program adding prestige.

Today, that hierarchical arrangement has changed, and the most common trend is to eliminate the undergraduate program. There are numerous reasons why this option is appealing: (1) The baccalaureate degree is the most teacher-intensive and therefore the most expensive to offer. (2) The Pew Health Professions Commission (1995) recommend a focus on the graduate level in relation to predicted workplace jobs. (3) Graduate education is perceived as more prestigious.

There is some intercollegiate experimentation going on, mostly in programs articulated across different colleges and universities. Other programs are once again thinking about the doctoral degree as the entry program. Some explorations of this option a few decades earlier were less than successful. Accelerated programs are still popular, either to serve new types of adult learners entering nursing programs or simply to provide for quick entry to graduate education.

Decision points concerning which programs to offer include determining the scope of the school's program. Will the department attempt to educate all levels from baccalaureate to doctoral? Within the selected levels, what will be the scope of specialties or different programs available? One role or several? A school that attempts to do everything may find itself spread too thin. If there are too few applicants distributed over many programs, the cost of the faculty will rise and its efficiency will suffer. Many nursing departments are making program choices based on an analysis of available niches identified through consumer research.

In effect, all the changes have been directed away from the hierarchical model (associate-baccalaureate-master-doctorate) and toward the *boutique model,* in which a faculty picks and chooses which options will be offered and in what format. This change is entirely in keeping with an era that is dominated by strategic management and other resource-driven models. Selections based on specialty expertise and on which program will get the most mileage (in income and in prestige) are perfectly in keeping with these models. The models also hold to the consumer orientation whereby customers (in this case students) may pick and choose. Alternatively, the consumer is considered in advance, while the programs to be offered are selected. Market research is the tool in this case.

The Content of Programs

Within virtually all basic programs, whether baccalaureate or associate degree, the issue is how to convert from an acute care orientation to a comprehensive community care model. Originally, the combined non-acute types of care were called *distributive* care (Lysaught, 1981), a term we will use for simplicity here. By whatever name, most curricula today are adding elements of ambulatory, convalescent, chronic, and preventive-educative care. In some cases the vision is traditional, merely adding the old public health (community) models, including the determination of whether the individual or the population group is the appropriate target of such care. Other programs incorporate new slices of the nonacute pie, such as convalescent care or community-based case management.

Absorption of diverse kinds of nursing care, taking place in various and disparate settings, calls for yet another curriculum decision: whether the faculty will evolve a plan with courses that are "setting-neutral," or whether courses will be designed around the diverse settings and types of care. *Setting-neutral* refers to content devised to be applicable in any setting, from hospital to home care. The opposite design is to compartmentalize content according to the setting in which the given aspect of care is most likely to be delivered. Some programs use a combination of these two approaches. We do not yet have enough data on these new curricula to determine which strategy will prove to be more effective. However, we know that generalized knowledge is not as easy for students to apply in diverse settings as was once assumed.

Another major change in nursing programs that convert from an acute care focus to a distributive care model is the need to consider the many different clinical placements. New nonacute facilities must be identified and wooed, and roles must be negotiated for students participating in these settings. From the faculty position, there are both advantages and disadvantages in the distributive model. On the plus side, the model gives the faculty a wider choice of clinical options, and this is important in an era when the decreasing number of acute care beds increases the competition for acute care placements.

On the minus side, there is the problem of preparing beginners to function in environments where they may lack the continuous consultation with experts available in the acute care facility. This problem is accentuated when the responsible clinical faculty member has students in diverse community sites and cannot be physically present with each one at all times. To plan these new distributive programs effectively is no small matter. However, more and more books, such as Matteson's (1995) are becoming available, suggesting methods of curriculum conversion.

Faculties have had to rethink some of their most dearly held principles and practices in designing today's curricula. For example, under the pressure of adding content about more diverse care, some groups have tried to consolidate by creating a "core" course that abstracts principles applicable in all subsequent courses. The notion sounds simpler than it is, for core concepts frequently look quite different in different specialties. For example, the idea of adaptation applied in an acute cardiovascular focus is so different from the notion of adaptation in a well-care clinic that the faculty can hardly expect students to carry over learning.

Unfortunately, in the past this lack of carryover learning has often been a source of mistrust; faculty members accuse peers of failing to "teach" whatever principle was involved. This lack of trust may have been part of the origin of a procedure unique to nursing education: "team teaching," in which all team members attend the lectures of their peers. Obviously, this cost-inefficient method seldom survives in today's economy.

Core concepts can form the basis of a final capstone course. In this application, concepts that have diverse applications in different domains are examined jointly and synthesized as a final expression of learning.

Nursing curriculists have long been compulsive about "coverage," with a false notion that if a particular subject isn't covered in some course, there will be a major gap in the student's education. The irony is that this places a premium on someone's "speaking the words" in a class rather than on the student's understanding and retention. New curricula must have faith in the student's ability to make up for the omissions that will inevitably occur in a streamlined program. One method that is being tried extensively is to organize curricula around *process* rather than *content*. Hence, today's curriculum is heavy on tactics, strategies, so-called critical thinking skills, systems management, and processes of acquiring and retrieving information. Although this conversion to process is a popular answer, it is too new to have much supportive data as to its effectiveness.

We may find that the rush to teach critical thinking skills, for example, is no more successful than teaching someone how to drive a car without practice. It may be that critical thinking arises in the process of struggling through patient issues and cannot be separated out effectively as mere "content." This may turn out to be the same kind of error as attempting to teach the nursing process apart from its application. Contextual learning certainly seems to be the name of the game, as in Benner, Tanner, and Chesla's (1996) research. Indeed, we may find that "critical thinking practices," often appearing in books as added sections of a revised edition, may discourage students from seeing critical thinking as an inherent part of *all* their nursing deliberation and action. Every process element of a curriculum will have to be analyzed in terms of its effectiveness when removed from pertinent content for teaching purposes.

In the push for economy and efficiency, many curricula are consolidating courses, with the notion of "streamlining," that is, eliminating any possible redundancy. As we move into setting-dominant or setting-neutral curricula, there is a great need for such economy; but sometimes the methods used are just not effective, especially if they eliminate the contextual clues that make learning meaningful to students.

However nursing education is planned, its associate and baccalaureate levels are undergoing a serious conversion from being based on acute care to being based on distributive care. This means that virtually every basic curriculum nationwide is in the midst of reinventing itself. Although this adaptation represents a major curriculum change, it is hardly a decision point, because everyone is doing it.

Today, it may be that the greatest decision point occurs at the master's level when a faculty chooses which sorts of advanced practitioners to prepare: clinical nurse specialists (CNSs), nurse practitioners (NPs), or a combination of both. A preference has already been made in the job market and in the choices of prospective students. On both counts, the practitioner role is ahead. The issue for many faculties is whether to convert to NP education, whether to keep both CNS and NP tracks, how to convert, and how to get an appropriate practitioner faculty. As happens when everyone gets on the same bandwagon, the issue of oversupply of NPs looms on the horizon, as does the notion of how nursing will be affected when the practitioner role becomes the typical graduate-level role.

The NP role is complex, particularly in its articulation with medicine. One can look at the NP role as a link providing for rapprochement with medicine, something to be highly desired in an era when cooperative care has clearly replaced isolated functions for each profession. This rapprochement occurs because the MD and the NP speak the same language and share many of the same goals. Indeed, physicians were usually the faculty in early NP programs, and sometimes they retain that teaching function even today. Most NP programs are designed on what approaches a medical model, that is, with a focus on pathology, diagnosis, and pharmacotherapeutics. With this similarity to medicine, the NP role may improve the relations between the two professions in the educational facility and in community workplaces. In long-standing working relationships, parity develops between MDs and NPs, resulting in increased mutual respect, especially when the NP is an equal in the practice and has similar rights, privileges, and obligations.

Alternatively, when the work situation is such that NPs are being used to replace more costly physicians, the role may become a source of friction to MDs rather than a link between professions. The trend toward substitution is encouraged under managed care because of economics, and nurses are the distinct "winners," albeit at the cost of good relations with physicians who see themselves losing jobs. On the whole, the issue of NPs against MDs or side by side with MDs is mixed at this time.

Another contemporary masters-level decision calls for a choice between the more traditional mainstream curriculum (usually with a dominant physiological basis and a medical model) and the newer holistic curriculum. By *holistic,* I mean a theory that disdains any form of reductionism and is heavy with "new age" therapies such as therapeutic touch, guided visualization, and meditation. Because these programs arise from radically different philosophies of nursing, it is difficult to combine both philosophies under one roof, although several schools are doing just that. This issue of a medical model or a holistic model arises in both CNS and NP programs.

CHANGES IN THE FACULTY'S ROLE

All the changes in the collegiate administrative environment and in the nursing programs of study have had dramatic effects on the role of the nursing faculty. The nursing faculty member, like his or her peers in practice, is facing new demands for performance, and most of the demands relate to saving resources. Often this translates into a demand that each faculty member increase productivity, one way or another. The increase may be in: (1) number of students taught in classes, (2) the number of students taught in clinical practica, (3) number of courses taught per year, (4) the amount of external funding the faculty member is expected to bring in, or (5) the amount of faculty practice required.

The demands may be discombobulating to faculty members who have cut their teeth on the typical faculty life of earlier eras, that is, with enough role autonomy to more or less determine what they will or will not do. As in the practice setting, the days that seemed harried at the time are now viewed as the leisurely good old days. The truth is that these days are over except in the best-funded universities and colleges.

Even the cherished benefit of tenure is threatened in many programs. The security of tenure once offered in the name of academic freedom is threatened now, not because of what a faculty member believes or says, but because a faculty member is judged on the criterion of productivity.

Increased Class Size

Receiving credit for an increased number of students in a class may be the easiest adjustment for a faculty member. Certainly the teacher who primarily relied on the traditional lecture method will have fewer adjustments (though this is not to say that the method is to be preferred). There are effective ways, other than lectures, in which one may interact with larger groups. Nursing faculties have long had a love affair with teaching methods, and some of the preferred methods require considerable one-on-one interaction. We may need to abandon many of these methods in favor of one-to-group interactions.

Testing, of course, is complicated by increased class sizes. It is to be hoped that faculties will not entirely substitute multiple-choice examinations, which can be machine-graded, for student papers, essays, and written examinations, which are more likely to elicit critical thinking and communication skills. Nursing students clearly need to learn to compose their thoughts and commit them to paper, even if grading such work requires more time.

When it comes to increased class size, nursing has much to learn from medicine, which has handled large classes throughout its history. Indeed, interprofessional education, which benefits everyone, may have much to teach us about methods as well as content.

Increased Numbers of Students in Clinical Practica

Having accountability for more clinical students is a greater challenge for the teacher than is an increase in number of classroom students. The question of how one can closely monitor and evaluate numerous students, some at geographic distances from each other, has led to some interesting and productive collaborative models with practicing nurses. As noted earlier, some models satisfactory from the educator's viewpoint have been rejected by practice personnel because they shift the burden of clinical education to the practitioner.

Sometimes faculties attempt to overcome clinical practice problems by increasing off-unit hours for the students. This may involve lengthening preconferences and postconferences. This is a great disservice to the student. As we learn more about how students learn (Benner, Tanner, & Chesla, 1996), we understand that hands-on immersion in the clinical domain is the single most critical factor. Indeed, clinical time should be increased rather than decreased, despite the challenge that this may pose for the faculty member.

Distributive education is an extra burden on a faculty if students are placed at different sorts of agencies. When this happens, it is virtually impossible to guarantee that one student's education is comparable to another's. Clinical practice comes to be smorgasbord of samplings of experience rather than the older model in which clinical arenas were live laboratories where student were "checked out" in various required processes and procedures. Using the *smorgasbord model* instead of the *proving-ground model* means that accountability for graduate clinical skills is no longer the program's responsibility—an emergent notion that dismays workplace administrators.

Responsibility for an Increased Number of Courses

Many institutions are renegotiating the number of courses for which a faculty member has responsibility. Sometimes this involves changing prior contracts; sometimes it simply means an arbitrary order on an administrator's part. Although actual faculty cutbacks are still the exception, many institutions are using attrition to trim the size of their faculty. There is little question that an increase in the number of courses taught is a sharp demand for enhanced productivity.

Perhaps the greatest weakness here is that some teachers use student-led classes. This is a poor way to decrease the faculty's workload. Students know when they are being used, and the end result is always bad. Today's student is litigious, and the teacher cannot expect to shift accountability to an inexpert student without penalty. Students view themselves, not inaccurately, as consumers who are paying for someone else to educate them. A wise faculty will take this same consumer-oriented viewpoint. This is not to say that group methods and student's involvement are to be eschewed, only that they are not a substitute for the input of an expert, prepared teacher. The truth is that a faculty job involves more work these days, and not all of it will fit into regular on-campus work hours.

Demands for External Funding

Today, many faculty appointments are contingent on the faculty member's bringing grants with him or her. This may be problematic because (1) many grants are given to the institution rather than to the principal investigator, and (2) funding is very competitive. Funding organizations are getting more proposals because of the demands placed on faculty members. Competition for the fewer available grants is fierce. As with the rest of the nation, many grant funding sources are finding themselves in a cutback situation, making the acquisition of grants a major challenge for faculty members.

When a faculty member is hired without concomitant grants, it is often with the expectation that he or she will acquire funding within a specified grace period. Of course, the irony is that faculty members dependent on such "soft money" may hold positions that will be eliminated as soon as the outside funding dwindles. Nor is a faculty member likely to be retained if he or she fails to produce the promised funding.

If the demand for high-quality teaching along with high productivity sounds like managed care, it is no surprise. The expectation is identical: that one will maintain quality with decreasing institutional resources.

Faculty Practice

Faculty practice is a growing expectation in most schools. Indeed, faculty members' salary is often a negotiation between the organization where they practice and the one where they teach. Because practice salaries are typically higher than faculty pay scales, the combined salary is often to the faculty member's advantage. Of course, there are places where the school "sells" the faculty member's practice time and keeps the income for its own coffers. Financial distribution arrangements for money earned in practice may be found everywhere along this curve, favoring the faculty member or favoring the school. In general, faculty practice takes some of the financial heat off most schools because it enables faculty members to earn a larger salary without requiring the school to invest more money.

Finance alone, however, is not the reason for the demand that all faculty members practice. As care becomes increasingly complex, there is little room for the "general nursing teacher" (who may tend to become clinically outdated). This demand for updated clinical competence also marks the end of those traditional programs of nurse teacher education which had a lot of content about teaching methods and little upgraded clinical knowledge.

With the movement of so many clinical specialist master's programs to nurse practitioner programs, the demand for faculty members to have clinical competence becomes a mandate. Often they are expected to precept nurse practitioner students as they care for patients (or to call on their clinical practice colleagues to do the same).

SUMMARY

Nursing education today, like case management, is dominated by (1) combined goals of quality and cost savings; (2) an outcomes orientation; (3) a group, rather than an individual, mentality; (4) an interprofessional approach to teaching health care; (5) an expanding notion of the settings where care will be delivered; and (6) a consumer orientation (whether the consumer is the patient or the student). A resource-driven approach is compatible with these changes in education. A strategic management approach works well in the education setting. Many changes are a result of environmental factors and cost control. They have an impact on program choices and on the faculty's roles in equal measure. In each case, the perspective involves marketing, a consumer orientation, and increased productivity.

REFERENCES

Benner, P. A., Tanner, C. A., & Chesla, C. A. (1996). *Expertise in nursing practice: Caring, clinical judgment, and ethics.* New York: Springer.

Lysaught, J. P. (1981). *Action in affirmation: Toward an unambiguous profession of nursing.* New York: McGraw-Hill.

Matteson, P. S. (Ed.). (1995). *Teaching nursing in the neighborhoods: The Northeastern University model.* New York: Springer.

Pew Health Professions Commission. (1995). *Critical challenges: Revitalizing the health professions for the twenty-first century.* San Francisco: Author.

TEST YOUR UNDERSTANDING

Multiple-Choice
Select the one *best* answer.
1. *Why has the growth of nurse practitioner programs outpaced the growth of programs preparing clinical specialists?*
   a. Their novelty makes them popular among faculty members.
   b. Faculties want to serve the express needs of their communities better.
   c. Student enrollments are up for practitioner programs, down for clinical specialist preparation.

2. *What is the best way to describe the changing role of the nursing faculty? It is:*
   a. A change in content more than in amount of work.
   b. An increase in amount of work more than a change in content.
   c. Both a change in content and an increase in amount of work expected.

3. *What is the* chief *difference between the smorgasbord model (SM) of clinical experience and the older proving-ground model (PGM)?*
   a. SM loosens the prior PGM relationship between clinical experience and accountability for specific learning.
   b. SM allows for more diversity in clinical placement than PGM.
   c. SM requires more "in-place" preceptors than PGM.

4. *Why is the learning of "core" content often ineffective?*
   a. It is hard to identify core elements.
   b. Core is so basic that students have little interest in it.
   c. The same core concept may look quite different in different applications.

Discussion of Answers

1. a. Popularity among faculty members is not a factor; indeed, it is difficult for many schools to find enough people prepared to teach this role.
   b. It is true that a community may need more practitioners, but not all faculties base their curriculum choices on public demand yet.
   c. This is the correct answer.

2. a. The amount of work required has increased substantially.
   b. With the move to distributive education, much of the teaching content has changed.
   c. This is the correct answer.

3. a. This is the correct answer.
   b. The SM model does allow for more diversity, but this is not its chief difference from the PGM.
   c. Although in-place preceptors would be a great help in SM, they would also be useful in PGM.

4. a. Identifying core elements is not that difficult, so this is not the reason that the learning is ineffective.
   b. If students evince little interest in core, it is because its significance never seems clear, not because it is so basic.
   c. This is the correct answer.

11

The Educational Process: How Do We Achieve It?

Managed care, with its cost-control mentality, has affected nursing education in many ways. That changes in the health care environment have an impact on education is not surprising in an era when, as Pesut (1998) says:

> Significant shifts include the fusion of work and learning. The emerging value of perpetual learning that affects professional practice is replacing the current disconnection between academic and practice realities. (p. 37)

The most important impact in this interface is that education must respond to the demands of future employers that students be educated to function in the managed care system. Managed care imposes many new structures on health care, and a nurse who does not understand what is happening will surely be overwhelmed. Second, as was indicated in Chapter 9, models having structures congruent with managed care have infiltrated into the educational systems as well. Hence, the faculty member had better understand the underlying principles in order to understand the environment in which he or she works. This chapter will (1) explore how education applies its own models, structurally congruent with managed care models; and (2) review the process and problems of teaching relevant aspects of managed care to students.

NEW PRINCIPLES UNDERLYING THE TEACHING OF NURSING

Many principles of managed care have invaded the teaching of nursing, as one would expect in this era. Chief among them are: (1) a consumer orientation, (2) a value system based on quality plus quantity, (3) an outcomes orientation, 4) decision making based on group norms, and (5) team building. These aspects will be reviewed briefly as they apply in the educational setting.

Consumer Orientation

Not only do faculties need to meet new demands from cost-conscious administrations, but they face increasing demands from students as well. Like everyone else in the system, students have begun to assess what they get for their money. They seriously question what sort of education they are receiving for the steep tuition they pay. In other words, students are assessing their education from the perspective of a consumer, and that involves two elements: (1) the quality of the education, and (2) how the degree will benefit them.

QUALITY OF THE EDUCATION

The quality of teaching has become a serious issue; students who once silently resented a rehash of old materials now sue. Like their service colleagues, faculty members had better acquire a customer orientation, and that means pleasing the customer on two fronts: classes need to be interesting and need to present worthwhile new information. The student is no longer a passive participant in the educational process. He or she is in the driver's seat, exactly like the purchaser of a new car in relation to a salesperson. Schools and faculty members are expected to facilitate students' achievement, abandoning an orientation toward putting students through unnecessary hoops and obstacles.

The customer orientation has caused many changes in the education delivery system, such as these:

1. Convenient locations, including satellite and distance education aided by interactive television, computer-assisted instruction (CAI), and Internet courses.
2. Faculty members' teaching courses rather than focusing exclusively on their research while letting teaching assistants lecture.
3. Classes offered at times convenient for students, not necessarily for the faculty—one day a week, say, or on weekends and evenings so as to be compatible with work schedules.

Students not only demand better teaching but may sue if they don't get it, so a faculty member may be wise to couch the benefits and requirements of a course in contractual terms. Although this might have seemed like legalistic overkill only a decade ago, such requirements, spelled out within the course outline, offer both parties protection. Nor can the faculty member change the rules later—for example, by altering the basis for assigning course grades or by adding extra assignments.

Similarly, due notice should be given to a student who is failing. It is not acceptable simply to give a failing grade at the end of a course. Litigious students can and do make much of the failure to notify. The same principle applies on a grander scale when faculty members decide to terminate a student near the end of his or her program of studies. Unless it can be proved that the student was made aware of the possibility of failure throughout, the faculty may not only face a lawsuit but may lose it. Courses of study are highly expensive these days, and dismissing a student simply cannot be taken lightly—he or she has invested a small fortune in the education. Faculty members can no longer leisurely take a few terms to decide that a student doesn't measure up. A failing student must be spotted early in the program.

BENEFITS OF THE DEGREE

In prior eras, a nurse got an education (at least a graduate education) to get a better job. Now, nurses often get advanced degrees merely to hold on to their present jobs. Others turn to education as an alternative when they lose their jobs and cannot find equivalent new ones. Today's student shops for educational opportunities, making choices based on anticipated outcomes. Indeed, when degrees fail to produce the anticipated benefits, a school may find itself besieged by unhappy alumni.

Some of the most recent causes of disaffection have included preparing too many midwives (a popular specialty) for the needs of a local community, and preparing nurses with clinical doctorates in an area where there are no jobs. In the practice setting, for good or ill, nursing directors have frequently eliminated the roles of such well-prepared staff members as a strategy for saving costs. Under managed care, clinical specialists also find themselves consistently losing out to nurse practitioners in the hiring institutions. In some locations, even beginning graduates have difficulty finding jobs. It is important that the school be clear from the start about the actual status of the local employment market.

Quality Plus Quantity

Another major shift inherited from managed care is a radical change in the underlying concept of nursing—that is, seeing nursing as a blend of quality and quantity care. This blend has been the major principle stressed throughout this book. It is the same principle as one finds operating in managed care, and the new element is the additional demand for *quantity*, which one may translate as *productivity*. On graduation, the nurse will have a heavier work assignment than was the case in the past. In the midst of a hectic environment, nurses must be able to see through the forest of demands in order to make the best use of their time. Nurses must be taught how to prioritize and select the most important work when the environmental pressures are greater than the resources (often their time) at hand. If managed care is built on a balance of quality and cost control, so is the role of the individual nurse. This means that he or she must selectively deliver the most critical elements of care to a patient group with the most efficiency. Resource-driven care is one model that blends quality and quantity.

Outcomes Orientation

The outcomes orientation of managed care has affected the teaching of nursing in several ways. We can look at: (1) faculty outcomes, (2) student outcomes, and 3) patient outcomes as taught to students. Students (as well as faculties) need to learn to view outcomes as the criteria by which everything else is judged.

FACULTY OUTCOMES

Faculties are learning to view their success or failure in terms of students' learning. After all, if the student fails to learn, the rest is meaningless. Focusing on outcomes can be exhilarating; it frees the teacher to experiment with multiple teaching methods—whatever achieves the desired learning.

Many new teaching methods are designed to achieve the same learning outcomes more creatively (or in ways that increase students' involvement). Modern substitutes for classroom teaching include computer-assisted instruction (from simple programs to the most elaborate interactive video productions), Internet courses, and programmed learning packages (often assigned in continuing-education units). Most of today's assisted learning programs have their own testing mechanisms, allowing the learners to know what they have learned as the course progresses. Hence, the students keep track of their outcomes throughout the learning experience. These methods allow the learner to set his or her own pace because the timing is not controlled by a faculty member. Some learning laboratories have been designed so that students can videotape return demonstrations, submitting their final tapes, when they are ready, to the instructor for evaluation. Interaction with these newer formats is welcomed by most younger nurses, but may still produce stress for older learners, particularly if it involves computer technology.

Some teachers develop alternative learning packages so that their students can achieve the same outcomes via different routes, each student selecting the method that best matches his or her individual learning style. In a sense, this flexibility is the boutique concept applied to learning methods.

Self-selected options are typical of today's teaching philosophy. That is, that the students should function independently, availing themselves of optional learning formats and opportunities. The new expectation is that a student, to a great degree, will assume responsibility for his or her own educational outcomes. The role of the faculty becomes one of making those diverse formats and opportunities available and evaluating students' achievement. As Pesut says:

> The teaching role for faculty in twenty-first-century learning is likely to be deemphasized. New role for faculty will be learning-centric, not teaching-centric. In the context of twenty-first-century learning, faculty are architects, designers, mentors, navigators, evaluators and certifiers of mastery, network scholars, researchers, and agents of the learning franchise. (p. 37)

The faculty as a facilitator and evaluator of learning outcomes, however, is quite different from abandoning learning to the student.

STUDENT OUTCOMES

If faculty members are learning to view the student's *learning* instead of their own *teaching* as the desired outcome, so are the students. Students are assisted by receiving clear objectives from faculty members in advance of any course or clinical learning experience. As the system becomes less uniform (more clinical sites, more optional learning methods), it is essential that students keep their bearings by having the desired outcomes in mind. Historically, we can trace the changing emphasis on outcomes in both practice and education systems. Nursing practice accreditation, for example, has moved from a content orientation to a process viewpoint and now to an outcomes orientation. This change in perspective is reflected in the newest evaluation criteria used for practice facilities by the Joint Commission on the Accreditation of Healthcare Organizations (JCAHO). In education, the pattern was seen early in the Regents External Degree Program of the state of New York. This program had no campus and no courses. Instead, candidates for various nursing degrees were subjected to intensive testing to see if they knew and could apply the appropriate content. With this outcomes orientation—called, appropriately, *competency-based learning*—the idea was that it mattered little where or how the students learned, as long as they did learn.

PATIENT OUTCOMES

Practices and procedures taught to students are now conveyed simply as various means for achieving desired patient outcomes. The student is taught to be flexible in selecting from among the various methods. Indeed, achieving desired patient outcomes will probably require that the student use different methods in different settings. Students no longer learn the "one right way" to do anything. Every practice is modified on the basis of the context in which it is used, and it is ultimately judged by whether or not the desired patient outcome was achieved.

Clinical pathways are tools based on patient outcomes that also serve to keep the student's thoughts and performance closely tied to goals. Unattained patient outcomes (variances) must be evaluated and will then form the basis for altering the methods of care.

Decision Making Based on Norms

Both the outcomes orientation and the quantitative perspective push the nursing mentality toward looking at group norms for patients rather than taking the old focus on the patient's individuality. This is not to say that the individuality of the patient gets lost, simply that many decisions will be based on group data rather than on projected individual outcomes. Today's student will begin with patient norms in terms of average physiological recuperation times, average patient learning curves, and anticipated emotional responses to a given situation—to name only a few of the norms that are used. Instead of starting with a notion that the patient is unique, the student judges the patient as a member of a given group (e.g., hip replacement) or a member of several groups (multiple diagnoses). Only then can the student consider how the patient might differ from the average case.

The vocabulary used today is telling. What was once a patient's *uniqueness* is now a *variance* from a projected clinical pathway outcome. Although faculty members may bemoan the impersonal character of today's system, they should also recognize how greatly it contributes to possible research and to the related development of care protocols. If one wanted to make another contrast with past eras, one could say that the system is deemphasizing the *art* of nursing in favor of the *science* of nursing.

The nursing student in any program, from beginning to doctoral, is taught to think in terms of average patient group outcomes. Norms dominate in the management of care, and the degree of tolerance for variance is a matter to be considered in every instance. For example, many nursing organizations hold that there should be zero tolerance for errors and accidents involving care. Alternatively, benchmarking works at improving one's outcomes rather than aiming at perfection, whether one is competing against one's own prior record or the record of competitors. Benchmarking, like other concepts in managed care, keeps its eye on the target.

Team Building

Today, *team building* does *not* refer to a return to "team teaching." Indeed, many applications of team teaching represent the most inefficient method of teaching in the history of nursing education. Instead, *team building* refers to teaching the nursing student to function as part of a multidisciplinary care team.

As noted earlier, the present era differs from past eras in which nursing tried to account for patient outcomes that could be attributed exclusively to nursing care. An insular view of nursing may have been necessary in the past when nursing was striving to establish itself as a unique profession with its own body of knowledge and its own theories; however, this view is no longer adequate. In fact, we need to consider whether our exclusive theories of nursing do us a disservice in our relationships with other players, especially physicians. Where outcomes are attributable to the combined work of many professionals, one could argue that it makes little sense for each group to approach the cooperative venture from a different theory.

The new viewpoint requires more complex practice, for the nurse must have a better understanding of what each health care worker on the team has to contribute to the patient outcomes. This shift to multidisciplinary care is reflected in the new JCAHO standards, which do *not* break desired outcomes apart on the basis of *who* achieves them. The new educational efforts to draw health professionals from various disciplines together in classes and courses, as well as clinical experiences, adds to their strength in team building and in working on a multidisciplinary team.

The case manager in a practice setting typifies the new mix of (1) an outcomes orientation and (2) goals achieved by the combined efforts of diverse professionals. Team building requires an approach that includes (1) knowing what other professionals bring to the table, (2) communication skills, and (3) assertiveness; and all these elements must be taught to, or inculcated in, students. Nurses usually have a good idea, for example, of what a physician contributes to a team, but they may be sadly lacking in knowledge of what a social worker or dentist might contribute. It is, of course, essential that the nurse learn to function as a full member of the team. Indeed, the leadership of a multidisciplinary team should shift periodically, depending on the problem being tackled. This means that the nurse must be prepared to assume team leadership when the problem addressed can benefit most from a nursing orientation. No amount of class time on the subject of team building will replace actual team experience for the student, and today's education should give the student numerous exposures to interdisciplinary work.

THE PROBLEM OF HOW MUCH IS TO BE LEARNED

A pedagogical problem created by the advent of managed care is that it adds so many new factors to what a nurse should learn. Take, for example, the excellent article by Huston and Fox (1998) in which they identify the 10 most important recent trends in nursing and their curricular implications. Most of these trends relate directly or indirectly to managed care. For instance, they list (1) economics as a driving force, (2) a continued movement of health care away from acute care hospitals, (3) growth in managed care, and (4) replacement of registered nurses with unlicensed assistive personnel (pp. 109–114).

If one looks at the curricular *additions* suggested by the authors for just these four (out of 10) trends, one finds the following items that might be considered new (or applied in an entirely new context): a shift to community-based experience; ability to communicate assessments to a multidisciplinary health care team; team training; information management for prevention; health education; political reform; cultural sensitivity; safety; communication with third-party payers; nature of home health care and community-based practice; health care reform; primary care nursing skills; upgraded physical assessment skills; client teaching; health supervision; family dynamics; principles of interviewing and coaching; case management; evidence-based practice, to provide information to insurers and regulators; health care finance and reimbursement; acronyms (PPO, PSO, ISN, IPA, HMO) and their implications for health care delivery; quality control mechanisms; audits (structure, process, and outcome); assertiveness; patient advocacy; principles of delegation; and ability to deal with cost-benefit and cost-effectiveness models.

Remember that these items are only those identified for *four* out of *ten* identified trends. The length of the list might be laughable except for the fact that the authors are correct: the new graduate needs knowledge of all these factors in order to survive in today's health care environment.

The point being missed here is the question of where all this added content will fit into a curriculum in which the clinical content (not addressed here) also grows more complex and extensive daily. This issue of expanding content is one with which nursing as a profession has not dealt adequately. It is enlightening to look at what happened in past eras when large numbers of nurse educators felt that the amount of content to be covered had gotten out of hand.

Abdellah, Beland, Martin, and Matheny (1960) were the first to offer a solution when the body-systems, disease-oriented curriculum model grew too extensive because of yearly additions in the form of new medical conditions and treatments. Using their research, Abdellah and her colleagues offered a new basis for a nursing curriculum: approaching it through problems that the patient presents to the nurse for resolution. Abdellah's own 21 nursing problems became the best known of the suggested approaches in this short but groundbreaking book. The initial method offered was far from orderly, confusing nursing and patient problems, but the content problem was well on the way toward resolution: curricula could be based on problems unique to nursing, rather than mimicking the format of medicine.

Out of these efforts grew at least two notions of problems—nursing problems (such as fluid and electrolyte imbalance) and patient problems (such as pain). Whatever path faculties took subsequent to the efforts of Abdellah and her colleagues, the orientation was away from diseases and conditions, and toward nursing and patient problems. With this solution, it no longer mattered if a new disease or condition were discovered. The student could apply the problem list to it; it need not be added as one more element in an already crowded curriculum. In essence, the student was given a new structure by which to intellectually organize the profession, one in which new information could be organized for the whole extent of a career.

Another approach to the problem of expanding content was evinced in various attempts, over the years, to move basic nursing to the doctoral level of education. This longer program would give the basic student all the time needed to learn the essentials. The problem with this solution was that few students were interested. For the investment of five or more years of study that these curricula required, most students felt that another career choice would be wiser. One can explain the general failure of the doctoral plan for basic nursing education in terms of a cost-benefit model. Nursing simply is not seen by first-time students as having a big enough payoff for that much initial investment of time and money. Later, once invested in the profession, nurses are more willing to look at extra years of study—but only if it gives them advanced, not basic, credentials.

The "crowded curriculum" again reared its head in the late 1970s, when a commission supported by the W. K. Kellogg Foundation looked at the issue anew. The National Commission for the Study of Nursing and Nursing Education, directed by Jerome P. Lysaught (1981), came up with a unique solution: nursing was simply too big for one profession. It should be divided in half according to its environmental setting, with nurses licensed for one or the other option: episodic (acute, hospital care) and distributive (community care). The professional nursing community received the Lysaught report with less than enthusiasm, and nothing more was ever done to move in this direction.

Looking at this model anew is most interesting, because we are in another era when context (environment) is critical. Indeed, because of the present shift toward community care, we are again in the full flush of the problem Lysaught and the commission tried to resolve. Once more, we have our heads in the sand concerning the breadth of knowledge needed in nursing. Once again, we assume that the nursing student should learn everything about both acute and nonacute care.

Do we need a new commission to address the problem of expanding content? Do we admit that it *is* a severe problem? Or do we continue to assume that faculties will teach "everything"? For education to avoid this problem is equivalent to the service sector's holding out for the model of total patient care. In both cases, a goal-directed model, impractical or not, is being used, rather than a resource-driven model.

The problem in education, as it was in service, is that the add-on strategy reaches a point where it is absurd. We are probably at this point now—as one infers from reading Huston and Fox's article. Obviously, Lysaught's solution of forming two professions could once again be considered, but it probably missed its historical chance.

It would be ideal for leaders from all of nursing (practice and education) to come together and deliberate on how to handle the problem. At present, each side holds the other culpable for failures. Practice leaders demand that new graduates be ready to function fully in any setting to which they are assigned. Unlike their forerunners in better-funded eras, today's practice leaders have no funds to pay for in-house internships for new graduates or to hire overlapping staff for a new nurse's time in orientation. On the other side, educators insist that they do not prepare students for actual jobs. Indeed, the smorgasbord model of clinical experience (just a sampling, not a proving ground) reinforces this claim. By default, educators win this battle, simply because they have their hands on the students last.

One approach to shared decision making might be to reexamine the difference between education and inculcation as learning tools. Briefly, education has to do with conveying information and teaching know-how. Basically, education cures ignorance and nothing else. Inculcation, on the other hand, develops in the person the patterns and folkways of a given culture—and nursing is clearly a culture. It is not something one learns as content, but the "ways and means" that one picks up from others in the environment. One is inculcated in the aspects of doing and being. These things are "caught" more than taught. Often the inculcated behaviors and values are not even discussed; they are simply accepted and acted upon.

Education at present is being held accountable for doing both tasks: education and inculcation; and it does a particularly poor job of the latter. One reason that faculties fail to inculcate nursing values and folkways is that faculty members are not practicing nurses. For many years the profession adopted the position that only faculty members would teach students in clinical arenas. Yet it is the student's goal to become a caregiver, not an educator. To learn the mores and folkways of a faculty member, rather than a caregiver, is to visit a nearby tribe. To learn from a practicing nurse, who is doing what one hopes to do upon graduation, is visiting the right tribe—the only effective route to inculcation into a culture and a value system. The use of practice preceptors was one of the best movements in nursing. Yet, as we said earlier, many practicing nurses are resigning from preceptorships because of the burdens placed on them in their own practice roles.

Practicing nurses and educators might start addressing the crowded curriculum by looking at which factors could be left for job inculcation and which factors are truly educational. Some but not all of the new demands (as identified by Huston and Fox), might be seen as items to be learned through inculcation rather than taught in an educational program. This is not to say that educational problems may be solved by passing them along to the service side. "Passing the buck" is a makeshift solution at best.

Instead, we might look at how the concept of inculcation relates to the nursing culture in which graduating students find themselves. Exactly what culture is absorbed from the work environment? We may find that the reason new nurses are confused has to do with a lack of cultural clarity rather than a lack of education. It may be that the values and the ways of coping in the workplace are shifting, uncertain, and confused. When one cannot figure out why the tribe acts one way and not another, it is no wonder that students fail to adapt and then, in turn, add to the confusion. Patterns must be clear before one can be inculcated into them. A sincere exploration of the nursing culture, with a view toward seeing how new graduates are inculcated into the workplace, might be productive.

Nor are faculties entirely excluded from all aspects of inculcation. For example, when faculties assume that nursing is based on economics as a driving force, that health care is moving away from acute care hospitals, that managed care is dominant and growing, and that use of group norms is an appropriate basis for planning patient care, then they are painting a picture of an environment and the ways in which nursing is to be conducted within that environment.

The convenient thing about inculcated aspects of learning is that they do not require teaching time; they are simply "caught" or assumed in the environmental context. For example, in earlier generations, we worried about students' being inculcated in an attitude of caring. A sense of caring, as we all know, can be caught far better by observing a caring nurse than by hearing a lecture on the principle of caring. And that observation can occur coincidentally while the student goes about his or her work—that is, it takes no additional time. Similarly, if a student presents to a faculty an overinvolved plan for teaching post–myocardial infarction patients, the teacher can simply tell this student to go back and consider the economy of time. This beats a lecture on the thrifty use of resources. We can streamline a curriculum, then, by differentiating those aspects that must be taught as specific content from those that are better conveyed through inculcation.

We are entering an era that presents us, once again, with a problem of curricular overcrowding. We might use the very tools of managed care to approach the problem: cost-benefit analysis, cost-effectiveness assessment, a resource-driven model of analysis, and a context-dominant explanatory model. At present, the problem of too much content sits on our doorstep unresolved.

SUMMARY

Managed care has an impact on nursing education in numerous ways. First, the curriculum should contain the basics of managed care in order for students to come to know the system in which they will be working after graduation. Second, philosophies, principles, and structures like those of managed care have infiltrated the educational environment. These include: (1) a consumer orientation, (2) a value system based on quality plus quantity, (3) an outcomes orientation, (4) decision making by use of group norms, and (5) team building.

The managed care system as a whole affects education of nurses by imposing a large amount of new content to be absorbed in all curricula, from basic to graduate. At present this increased demand for extra content has yet to be satisfactorily resolved. The needed learning will have to take place, either in school programs or in practice settings, and the obvious approach would call for both sides to plan together how to best meet this new demand.

REFERENCES

Abdellah, F. G., Beland, I. L., Martin, A., & Matheney, R. V. (1960). *Patient-centered approaches to nursing.* New York: Macmillan.

Huston, C. J., & Fox, S. (1998). The changing health care market: Implications for nursing education in the coming decade. *Nursing Outlook, 46*(3): 109–114.

Lysaught, J. P. (1981). *Action in affirmation: Toward an unambiguous profession of nursing.* New York: McGraw-Hill.

Pesut, D. J. (1998). Twenty-first-century learning. *Nursing Outlook, 46*(1): 37.

TEST YOUR UNDERSTANDING

Multiple-Choice

Select the one *best* answer.

1. *Which curriculum item is not an outgrowth of the era of managed care?*
   a. A consumer orientation toward students.
   b. A focus on both student and patient outcomes.
   c. Team teaching.

2. *Which of the following is not a principle to be applied to today's nursing education?*
   a. Use of normative data.
   b. Exclusive focus on qualitative data.
   c. Dominance of the value of efficiency.
   d. An outcomes orientation.

3. *Which item could be conveyed by inculcation instead of education?*
   a. Taking pride in one's work.
   b. Deciding which patient to assess first.
   c. Determining which tasks could be omitted on an overly busy day.

4. *Which strategy reflects outcomes management applied to nursing education?*
   a. Multidisciplinary team building.
   b. Team teaching.
   c. Competency-based education.

Discussion of Answers

1. a. Remember that this is a *negative* question. A consumer orientation is directly related to managed care through marketing and institutional competition, among other considerations.
   b. Outcomes management is at the heart of case management and clinical pathways in managed care.
   c. This is the correct answer.

2. a. This also is a *negative* question. Today we are in an era when normative data are the basis for most care planning.
   b. This is the correct answer.
   c. Efficiency is an important measure of cost; as such it is very important.
   d. An outcomes orientation is dominant today.

3. a. This is the correct answer.
   b. This requires specific knowledge about patients' cases; hence it involves education.
   c. This requires specific knowledge about the importance of various therapies; hence it involves education.

4. a. Team building is part of managed care, but it is not based directly on outcomes.
   b. Team teaching is based not on outcomes but on coordinating teaching efforts.
   c. This is the correct answer.

Index

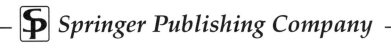

S Springer Publishing Company

Developing Research in Nursing and Health
Quantitative and Qualitative Methods

Carol Noll Hoskins, PhD, RN, FAAN

"It is a clear and unencumbered 'snapshot' of essential information that can serve as a study guide for graduate students, a handy reference for researchers and faculty, and an 'instructor's manual' for teaching research. I would certainly use this guide...."
—***Harriet R. Feldman,*** *PhD, RN, FAAN*
Dean and Professor, Pace University Lienhard School of Nursing

This handy volume is an excellent adjunct to traditional research texts and courses, and a boon to educators and researchers challenged to "know all" about the processes of research. Some of the important general features include:

- an outline format designed to highlight key information
- clarification of confusing and difficult information
- exemplars used throughout each chapter and in the appendices

This valuable guide stands out from traditional texts by offering a succinct overview of key sources of nursing and related literature; differentiation of the theoretical framework of quantitative and qualitative studies; a guide to abstracting research studies; clear presentation of the types, rules, and procedures of sampling; and a conceptual appproach to organizing descriptive and inferential statistics and qualitative data analysis.

Contents: Research in Nursing • The Research Question —- Hypotheses • The Literature Review, Definition of Terms, and Theoretical Framework • Research Designs • Sampling in Qualitative Designs—-Basic Issues and Concepts • Data Analysis and Interpretation—-Qualitative Designs • Principles of Measurement • Development of Quantitative Measures

1998   130pp   0-8261-1185-8   softcover

536 Broadway, New York, NY 10012-3955 • (212) 431-4370 • Fax (212) 941-7842

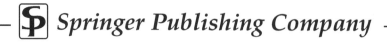 *Springer Publishing Company*

Integrating Community Service Into Nursing Education
A Guide to Service - Learning

Patricia A. Bailey, EdD, RN, CS
Dona Rinaldi Carpenter, EdD, RN, CS
Patricia Harrington, EdD, RN, CS

Service learning gives nurse educators a simple tool for linking classroom learning to the community. A growing movement among educators nationwide, it combines community volunteer service with a structured learning experience which includes student preparation and reflection. This book is a guide to applying service learning to the nursing curriculum, written by nurse educators who have created and implemented a successful program at the University of Scranton. It includes essays by community agency adminstrators who have participated in these programs, student feedback, and many case examples.

An indispensable aid for nurse educators engaged in preparing future health care practitioners for practice in community settings.

Contents:

- The Concept of Service Learning, *Dona Rinaldi Carpenter*
- Integrating Service Learning into the Curriculum,
  Patricia A. Harrington
- Critical Reflection, *Patricia A. Bailey*
- The Promises and Problems of Service-Learning,
  Dona Rinaldi Carpenter and Patricia A. Harrington
- Community Partnerships in Service-Learning,
  *Patricia A. Bailey, with personal stories by Peggy Begley,
  Janet Moskovitz, Tracy Lyn Svalina & Candal B. Sakevich*

1999   152pp (est.)   0-8261-1268-4   *hardcover*

536 Broadway, New York, NY 10012-3955 • (212) 431-4370 • Fax (212) 941-7842

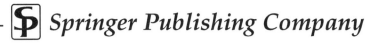 *Springer Publishing Company*

Evaluation and Testing in Nursing Education

Marilyn H. Oermann, PhD, RN, FAAN
Kathleen B. Gaberson, PhD, RN

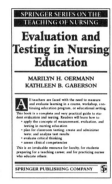

This comprehensive graduate level text is a valuable resource for nursing teachers, students, and health professionals involved in evaluating staff and developing protocols. The topics are organized into five broad areas: concepts of measurement, evaluation, and testing; test construction and analyzing; clinical and performance evaluation; interpreting and reporting test results; and evaluating educational programs.

Theoretical yet practical, **Evaluation and Testing in Nursing Education** features helpful models for improving the process, including numerous examples of test questions, and competency systems in health care settings.

Intended for use as a main text by graduate nursing students and as a handy reference for faculty, this book will also serve all health professionals concerned with efficient staff development.

Contents: Evaluation, Measurement, and Educational Process • Qualities of Effective Measurement Instruments • Planning for Classroom Testing • Objective Test Items: True-False, Matching, and Short Answer • Objective Test Items: Multiple-Choice and Multiple-Response • Essay Test Items and Evaluation of Written Assignments • Evaluation of Problem Solving, Decision Making, and Critical Thinking: Context-Dependent Item Sets and Other Evaluation Strategies • Assembling and Administrating Tests • Scoring and Analyzing Tests • Clinical Evaluation • Clinical Evaluation Methods • Social, Ethical, and Legal Issues • Interpreting Test Scores • Grading • Program Evaluation • Total Quality Management and Nursing Education

1998   336pp   0-8261-9950-X   hardcover

536 Broadway, New York, NY 10012-3955 • (212) 431-4370 • Fax (212) 941-7842

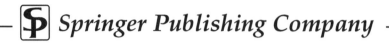
Springer Publishing Company

Clinical Teaching Strategies in Nursing

Kathleen B. Gaberson, PhD, RN

Marilyn H. Oermann, PhD, RN, FAAN

This practical book examines concepts of clinical teaching and provides a comprehensive framework for planning, guiding, and evaluating clinical learning activities for undergraduate and graduate nursing students and health care providers in a variety of settings.

Contents:

- A Philosophy of Clinical Teaching
- Outcomes of Clinical Teaching
- Preparing for Clinical Learning Activities
- Models of Clinical Teaching
- Process of Clinical Teaching
- Ethical and Legal Issues in Clinical Teaching
- Choosing Clinical Learning Assignments
- Self-Directed Learning Activities
- Learning Laboratories
- Simulations and Games for Clinical Learning
- Case Method, Case Study, and Grand Rounds
- Clinical Conference and Discussion
- Written Assignments
- Using Preceptors as Clinical Teachers
- Clinical Teaching in Diverse Settings

1999   320pp (est.)   0-8261-1278-1   hardcover $39.95 tentative

536 Broadway, New York, NY 10012-3955 • (212) 431-4370 • Fax (212) 941-7842